Praise for Gwen Lawrence

"Gwen has been the yoga coach for the New York Giants all of the years I've been in the franchise. Our players flock to her sessions to improve their flexibility, balance, and breathing awareness. She has had a tremendous impact on our performance enhancement."
—Bill Sheridan, Assistant Coach, New York Giants

"I have worked with Gwen for only a couple of months and I have recognized tremendous gains in my flexibility, core strength, and balance which are essential to staying healthy and explosive. I consider myself lucky to have learned as much from Gwen as I have in such a short time."
—Kevin Booth, Offensive Guard, New York Giants

"The Yankees have utilized Gwen Lawrence's services as an alternative way of providing the core stabilizations program of our players through her system of Power Yoga for Sports. I have found her to be extremely professional and look forward to working with her more."
—Brian Cashman, Senior Vice President and General Manager, New York Yankees

"Gwen is great. She *always* makes you feel like you can do it!"
—Hoda Kotb, television news anchor and co-host of NBC's *Today* show

"Gwen Lawrence has been a personal friend of mine for over 10 years. She has developed a unique profession that utilizes the best from the worlds of yoga and massage therapy. She combines conventional stretching, strength, and balance training with the teachings of mental discipline and breath awareness, all of which are so vital in the world of professional athletics."
—Frank Gifford, NFL Hall of Famer

"We have been a client of Gwen Lawrence's for 12 years and cannot give her a stronger recommendation. She has given us a tremendous boost in taking care of our various aches and pains and sports injuries over the years."
—Joy & Regis Philbin

"Gwen Lawrence has been a trusted friend for many years. More than just a friend, she has helped me maintain my health and rehab me through surgeries and injuries. Without a doubt, she is one of the finest teachers and practitioners in the whole country. Gwen Lawrence can change your life."
—Regis Philbin, television personality and host of "Live! with Regis and Kelly"

"We have worked with Gwen and her Power Yoga for Sports system for years and have found not only her style, but also her methods, to be as approachable as the girl next door. Far from scaring anyone off, Gwen's teachings make the practice of yoga something that anyone can do, at any time."
—Lee Woodruff, author of *In an Instant* and contributing reporter for "CBS This Morning"

"You have prepared me for everybody and anybody. There is nothing I can't do that they ask of me, and I know how to listen to them explain what they want. Thank you for teaching me how to grow confident in my own body! This is an immeasurable gift!"
—Christina Mason, competitive squash player

Body Sculpting with Yoga

Gwen Lawrence

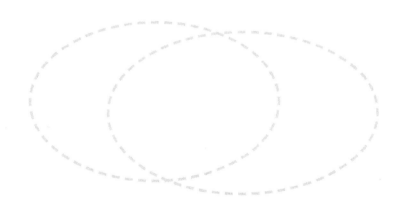

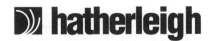 **hatherleigh**

hatherleigh

Hatherleigh Press is committed to preserving and protecting the natural resources of the earth. Environmentally responsible and sustainable practices are embraced within the company's mission statement.

Visit us at www.hatherleighpress.com and register online for free offers, discounts, special events, and more.

Library of Congress Cataloging-in-Publication Data is available upon request.
ISBN: 978-1-57826-526-8

Cover and Interior Design by Heather Magnan

Clothing provided by lululemon athletica® (www.lululemon.com) and Under Armour® (www.underarmour.com)

Printed in the United States
10 9 8 7 6 5 4 3 2

Contents

Dedication

I completely dedicate this book and its inspiration to the love of my life
My husband

My one and only
Who does everything
So I can pursue
My life
My dreams
My purpose

M.E.
&
B.T.C.

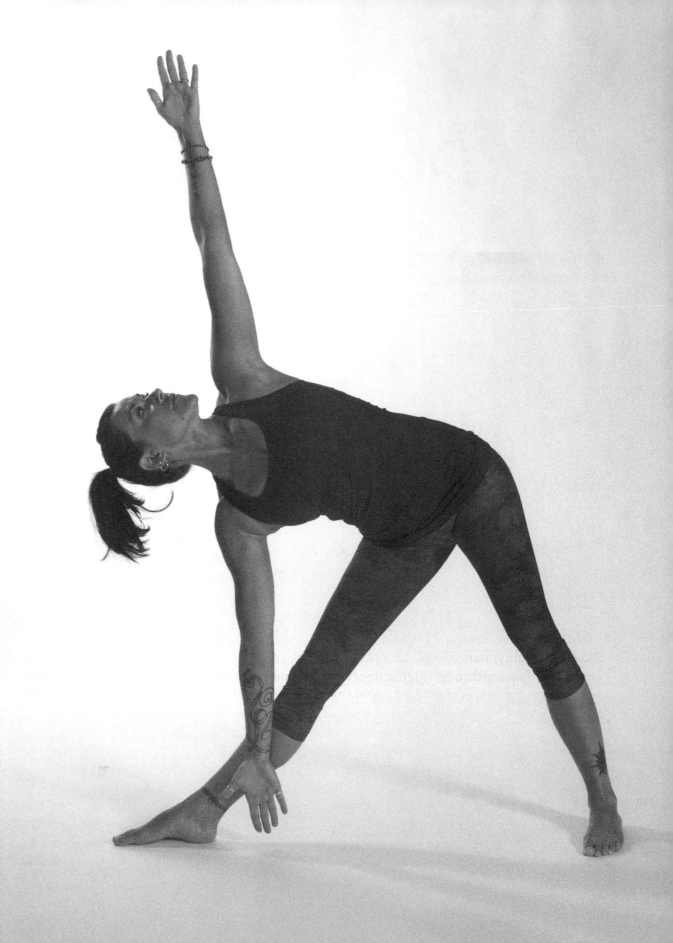

Introduction

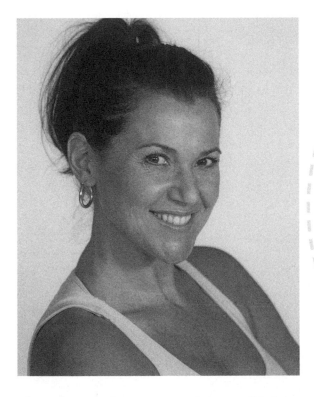

Gwen Lawrence, fitness professional and creator of the Power Yoga for Sports training program and the VYX™ (Vinyasa Yoga Extreme) system.

I have been a dancer since the age of 3. It was a world far different from the current *Dance Moms* mentality; dance kept me on the straight and narrow, committed and organized. I continued dancing through high school as a principal contributor and leader of the company. My dance teacher was strict and crystal clear on her objectives. At the time, I resented her style, but I now realize her approach was the seed that spawned my no-nonsense, tough love approach to teaching yoga to high-level athletes today, so thank you, Mrs. Kopp. My love of dance continued through college as my minor and eventually set the stage for my love of movement and my ability to choreograph the original body sculpting yoga flow series that are found in this book.

I have been a working fitness professional since the age of 18. I placed fourth in Miss Fitness America when I was in college and have always loved the feeling of lifting weights and cross-training my body. I worked and ran fitness facilities and created programs to help people reach their fitness goals. I even trained in step aerobics until the minute my first son was born. It is not surprising that he loves fitness and thrives on working out as all my sons do…they were exposed in utero!

After college I attended The Swedish Institute College of Health Sciences in New York City and have been a massage therapist to the stars and elite athletes since 1990. With massage, I have worked with physical therapists, in fitness facilities, with chiropractors, and on doctor referral. All of this experience has given me a deep knowledge and understanding of how the body works and rehabilitates, and also how to train the body to maximize performance. To be a yoga teacher you are required to study only 20 hours of anatomy, yet I easily have 100 times that and growing. (I know this because I own a Yoga Alliance-accredited yoga school, Laws of Yoga School of Yoga, where I teach people to become yoga instructors!)

Finally, I have a unique ability to read bodies. I position my clients and athletes to analyze them for imbalances and symmetry that inevitably (if left unaddressed) will lead to injury. Leaving symmetry problems unresolved is like never rotating the tires on your car and then just driving and driving on the balding tire until it blows! I have people around the world sending me photos to analyze their posture, and I help to relieve some nagging mysterious pains. To me, it's all about preventing injury in the first place and enhancing performance thereafter.

What Can This Workout Do for You?

Many of you are likely busy and motivated women, overworked moms, or just someone looking to bring better health habits into their life. *Body Sculpting with Yoga* will show you how to achieve your health and fitness goals through the powerful sculpting, toning, and strength-building benefits of yoga-inspired exercises.

It is not my intention to scare or intimidate you about my life's work with professional athletes. Quite the contrary. I tell you my journey so you can rest assured that the exercises and workouts in this book have been built off of my time-tested techniques and will bring results.

In *Body Sculpting with Yoga*, I give you the basics of yoga and then bump it up with weights and repetitions, along with creative series, so even if you have never tried a yoga workout, you can still feel comfortable with this hybrid approach to training. I ask that you just do it! There are no excuses. The first step is reading this book and the next step is taking action. Set your goals, set your intention, and set your pace, then watch what happens. You'll notice increased energy levels, an improved body image, and better sleep. Be a doer, not a watcher, and redefine your purpose to achieve fitness goals you never thought possible]

Every day, I help people transform their lives from good to great, helping my clients reach their highest potential using my power yoga for sports philosophy to **A**ttain fitness, find **B**alance, **C**reate goals, and **D**efine personal happiness in work, school, family, and life the way only an intuitive yogi and seasoned mom can. Now let's get started building the body you've always wanted!

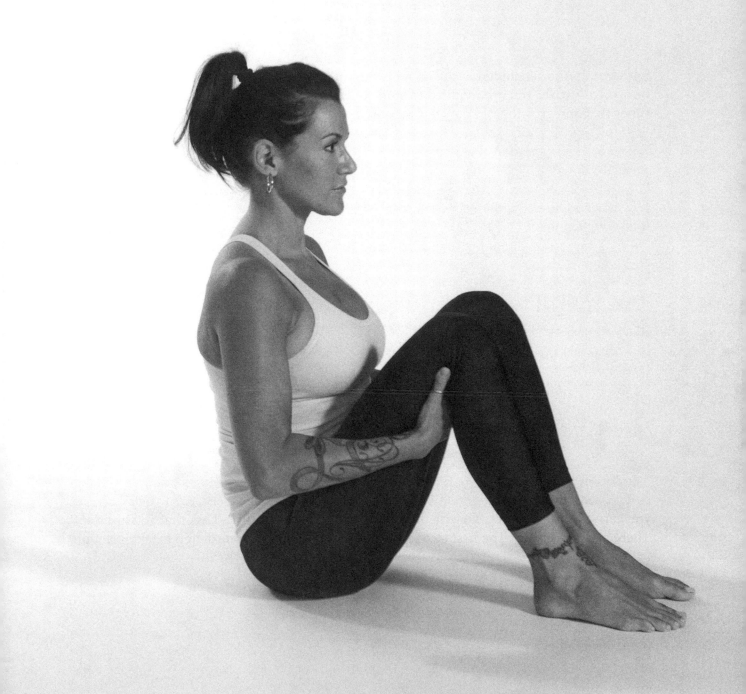

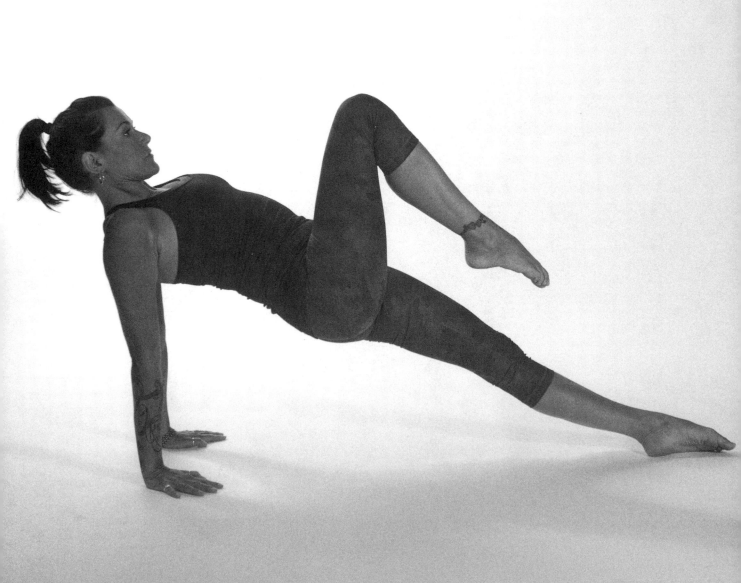

Part I:
Body Sculpting with Yoga

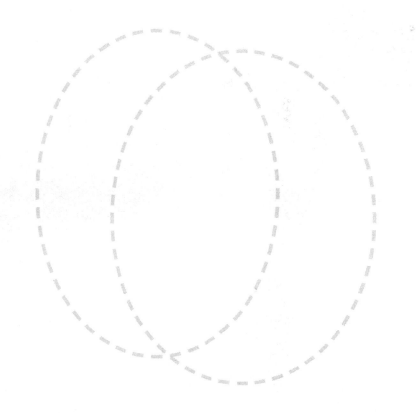

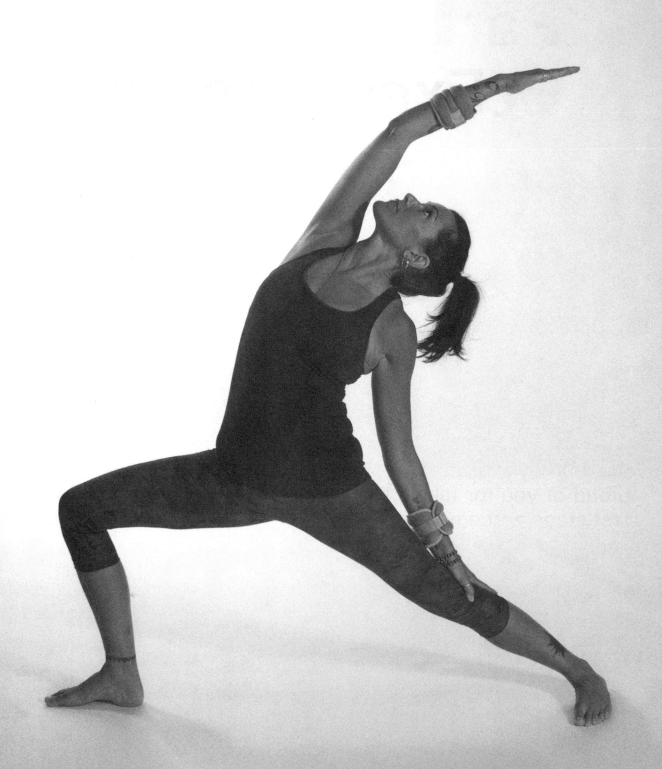

About the
Exercises

You have made the decision to move towards a better, healthier life and you are now ready to embark on this journey with me. I am so proud of you for taking the first steps and empowering yourself. Let's talk about the types of moves you will be doing and why, and also go over some do's and don'ts to expedite your results.

Types of Moves

Body Sculpting with Yoga utilizes an original hybrid yoga system that I developed, which takes the best aspects of my Power Yoga for Sports system, hybrid yoga, and VYX™ (Vinyasa Yoga Extreme).

The Power Yoga for Sports system caters to athletes of varying fitness levels, ranging from weekend warriors to professional athletes. The workouts are designed to enhance an athlete's performance and prevent injury by bringing awareness to their body and considering their training cycle, as well as utilizing specific yoga routines that are designed for the athlete's sport and position. All of this helps the athlete utilize their training time to the fullest. Power Yoga for Sports uses six training principles—balance, strength, flexibility, mental toughness, focus, and breathing—to get players to the next level.

Hybrid yoga is a type of yoga that incorporates the discipline and *asanas*, or poses, of traditional yoga and adds other training techniques such as weights, resistance bands, high-impact movement, jumping, plyometric-inspired moves, physio-balls, and much more to increase results and transform bodies. The focus of *Body Sculpting with Yoga* is to utilize the flow and physical benefits of yoga classes, while upping the game by adding traditional weightlifting moves and hybridized yoga poses that keep you engaged and moving.

The biggest challenge is utilizing VYX™ during your workout. This is a concept I trademarked, which involves attaching wrist weights and ankle weights, and even wearing a weighted vest, to increase the effectiveness of your most common yoga moves. By wearing the extra weight on your body, you get all the benefits that yoga has to offer coupled with the benefit of weight-resistance moves, which increases the difficulty, burns more calories.

With the combined benefits of the Power Yoga for Sports system, hybrid yoga, and VYX™, the *Body Sculpting with Yoga* workouts will:

- Increase bone density with resistance work
- Build muscle
- Burn more fat, even at rest
- Add cardio training to your yoga
- Keep you challenged and motivated
- Streamline your yoga training
- Speed up results

Types of Yoga

Ashtanga

Ashtanga is based on ancient yoga teachings, but it was popularized and brought to the West by Pattabhi Jois in the 1970s. It's a demanding style of yoga that follows a specific sequence of postures and links every movement to a breath. This is a sweaty, physically challenging practice.

Hatha

Hatha yoga is a generic term that refers any type of yoga that teaches physical postures. Hatha classes generally provide an introduction to the yoga postures and, depending on the teacher, can either be a basic or an advanced practice.

Hot Yoga

Hot yoga is performed in a heated room, similar to Bikram-style yoga. The difference between Bikram and hot yoga is that the hot yoga studio usually heats the room to 80-90°F and teaches whatever sequence they want. Bikram is specific to a 104°F room and teaches the same 26 poses in the same order for every class and teacher.

Iyengar

Iyengar yoga was developed and popularized by B.K.S. Iyengar. This is a very meticulous style of yoga, with utmost attention paid to finding the proper alignment in a pose. An Iyengar studio will stock a wide variety of blocks, blankets, straps, bolsters, and a rope wall.

Restorative

Restorative yoga is a way to relax the body and mind. Restorative classes use bolsters, blankets, and blocks to prop students in passive poses so that the body can experience the benefits of a pose without having to exert any effort. This is what I do with the New York Giants after every Monday night game.

Vinyasa

Vinyasa is the Sanskrit word for "flow," and Vinyasa classes are known for their movement-intensive practices. Vinyasa teachers choreograph their classes to smoothly transition from pose to pose, and often play music to keep things lively.

The Meaning of Yoga

Oxford Dictionary defines yoga as:

"A Hindu spiritual and ascetic discipline, a part of which, including breath control, simple meditation, and the adoption of specific bodily postures, is widely practiced for health and relaxation."

Simply put, yoga is the simplest form of non-judgment and brings together the connection between body, mind, and spirit through movement. With the hybrid approach to yoga found in *Body Sculpting with Yoga*, you can adjust your yoga routine to fit into your own life and get the most results in the least amount

Do's and Don'ts of the Body Sculpting with Yoga Workout

DO:

If working out on your own:

- Find a quiet space where you will not be disturbed

- Wear comfortable clothing that will allow movement

- Shut down your electronics to eliminate distraction

- Bring a mat and any other props you may nee

If taking a class:

- Arrive 10 minutes early

- Introduce yourself to your teacher and update them on any injuries, past and present

- Create your intention (what you wish to accomplish from the class that day)

- Be silent, so you can be more aware of your body

- Bring a towel, your own mat, and any props such as blocks or straps

- Wear comfortable and loose clothing

DON'T:

If working out on your own:

- Allow other people in the room with you

- Eat right before starting

- Rush through; take time for yourself

- Forget to drink water

If taking a class:

- Bring a cell phone or any other distraction

- Create expectations

- Arrive late

- Eat one to two hours before class (instead, eat lightly after class)

- Succumb to distraction

- Push through pain

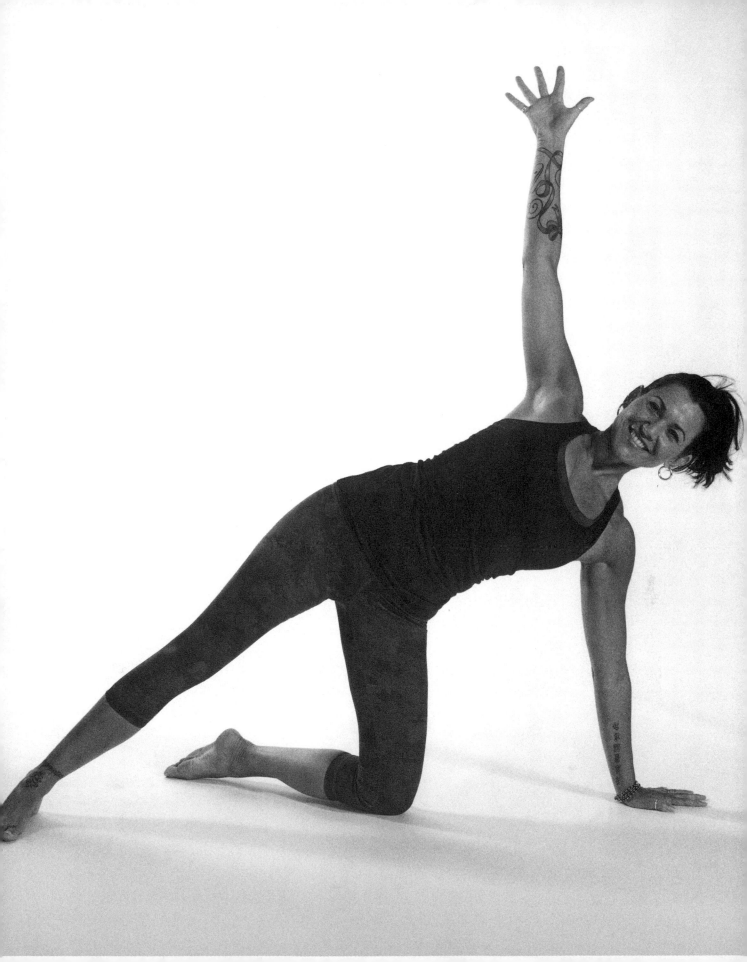

Body Sculpting

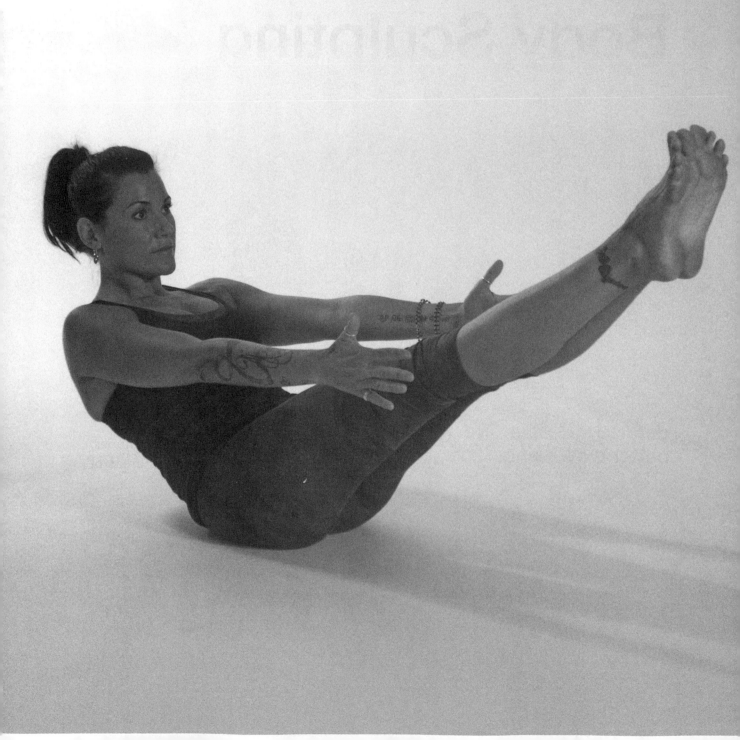

Benefits of
Body Sculpting
with **Yoga**

2

This chapter is meant to be an inspiration and motivator and will give you a better understanding of why yoga is important for injury prevention, more beautifully defined muscles, and overall better well-being.

Physical Benefits of Yoga

Yoga practice offers a wide variety of physical benefits, including:

- Enhanced flexibility
- Improved lubrication of joints
- Massaging the internal organs

- Body detoxification
- Weight loss
- Stress relief
- Toned and lean muscles
- Increased muscle mass

Enhanced flexibility: Continuous, systematic stretching on specific areas of the body will elongate and increase your flexibility over time. An effective flexibility-training program like the ones found in this book can increase your physical performance and effectiveness, improve the symmetry of your body, and help reduce your risk of injury by improving your range of motion. In addition, increased flexibility can lower tension on the back and spine and improve posture, which can help with breathing and oxygenation of the body. Stretching also increases the blood supply to your entire body (including muscle tissue), delivering essential nutrients through your blood stream.

Improved lubrication of the joints: Flexibility training improves performance because it helps to keep joints lubricated and healthy. Well-lubricated joints require less energy to move, so stretching can help you use your energy more efficiently. Stretching before a workout helps your muscles become more elastic, so they're better able to withstand the stress of exercise.

Massaging the internal organs: Bending, twisting, and moving the body in all directions literally massages your internal organs. This is beneficial because it helps in detoxing the body, so that you can focus on being fit.

Body detoxification: When you efficiently increase flexibility, lubricate the joints, and massage and detox the body, your body can function as it was intended. When you sweat, you help the body eliminate toxins, and when you twist and torque your body, you are wringing out the organs and skin and ridding your body of toxins. When you have a body in homeostasis it is more competent at shedding weight, sleeping to recover, and relieving and dealing with stress.

Weight loss: With the workouts in this book, you will increase your muscle mass with functional strength training, meaning that you use your body weight as resistance. In the advanced workouts you will add weights, which will increase your muscle mass even quicker. A body that has more muscle will be more efficient at burning calories and staying fit, even at rest.

Stress relief: Another important benefit of these yoga-inspired workouts is to relieve the detrimental effects of constant stress on the body. Our bodies are only meant to handle short bursts of stress. But with today's busy lifestyles, we are now constantly under varying levels of stress, and this endless stress has caused diseases and illnesses never documented before. When yoga instructors tell you to take a "healing breath," they aren't just using a metaphor. Recent studies show that practicing yoga and performing regular exercise may actually have a significant effect on a person's physiological well-being.

Toned and lean muscles: When most women set out to start a workout program it seems their end goal is a toned and lean body, not necessarily bulking up. The difference is to achieve an end point of toning, which requires combining strength training and stretching with fat burning.

Increased muscle mass: Improving your muscle mass is critical. A body with more muscle burns more fat, even at rest. In addition, you will get slimmer because 5 pounds of muscle takes up one-third less space on your body frame than 5 pounds of fat. So you may weigh the same but don't be fooled; you will be slimmer and a more efficient calorie-burning machine.

Mental and Emotional Benefits of Yoga

In addition to offering physical benefits, yoga also:

- Improves your ability to cope with psychological and mental difficulties
- Decreases anxiety and depression
- Boosts memory

Complementary Therapies in Medicine conducted a randomized trial to compare the effectiveness of yoga and relaxation as treatments for reducing stress and anxiety. This study compared the two treatment modalities at 10 weeks and 16 weeks to determine whether either modality improved stress, anxiety, blood pressure, and quality of life. Participants included 131 subjects with mild to moderate levels of stress. The participants did 10 weekly one-hour sessions of relaxation or yoga. The results following the 10-week intervention showed that stress, anxiety, and quality of life scores improved over time, and yoga was found to be as effective as relaxation in reducing stress and anxiety, and improving health. In fact, yoga was more effective than relaxation in improving mental health.

Improves your ability to cope with psychological and mental difficulties: Many mental health problems begin with physical stress and emotional stress that can trigger chemical changes in your brain. To prevent this, it can be helpful to reduce stress and restore normal chemical processes in your brain. Yoga and physical movement are great coping skills to enhance breathing and calm your body so that you are better prepared for your challenges.

Decreases anxiety and depression: The physical benefits of the poses in yoga aligned with the focused breathing is the perfect way to cope with symptoms of anxiety and depression. Calming the heart rate, lowering blood pressure, and easing respiration are concrete ways in which yoga helps with anxiety and depression.

Boosts memory: As we already mentioned, yoga helps reduce stress, and it has been discovered that people who experience constant levels of stress can literally damage and overload their brain. So by reducing stress, you are enabling your body to clear the head and allow it to focus on the things that are important for you to remember. In addition, inverted poses are a great way to bring a flush of blood and oxygen to the brain, which helps nourish the brain, keeps you more focused and clear, and improves neuromuscular functioning.

Transforming Your Body

The benefits of this hybrid yoga workout are exciting and real. Training with weights and yoga has been proven to increase HDL (good cholesterol), decrease LDL (bad cholesterol), lower high blood pressure, and reduce the risks of cardiovascular disease and diabetes. It also lowers the risk of breast cancer by controlling high estrogen levels linked to the disease, alleviates symptoms of PMS, and reduces stress and anxiety. Weight training and yoga also help to minimize the risk of developing osteoporosis by building bone mass.

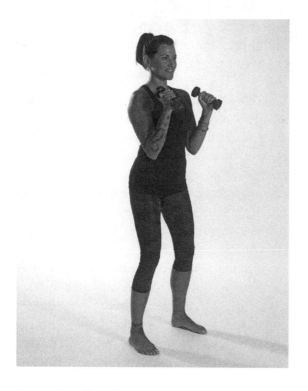

injury. Increased bone density and strength also reduces back pain and knee pain by building muscle around these areas. The way you sit and stand are influenced by a network of muscles in the neck, shoulder, back, and abdominals. When you create stronger bones with the musculature to support it, you will find that you can stand and sit straighter and more comfortably.

As you begin to notice these physical changes in your body, an amazing snowball effect happens. By combining the compelling benefits of yoga and weight training, the *Body Sculpting with Yoga* workouts will offer some amazing results in the way you look and feel. I am so thrilled for you to try this cross-training technique to excite you every day for six weeks to get you fit, cut, and healthy in a more holistic way.

Beyond all of these medical benefits, training with weights also offers many benefits to one's physical appearance, including increased muscle strength, power, endurance, and size, with enhanced performance of everyday tasks. You will be able to do everyday tasks like lifting, carrying, and walking up stairs with greater ease. The conditioning effect will result in firmer and more defined muscles. A boost in your metabolism (which means you will burn more calories when at rest) will reduce body fat, so you will gain muscle and lose fat. Over time you will notice decreases in your waist measurements and body fat measurements. If you are interested in becoming more athletic, you will be happy to know that using weights in your training will also result in strong muscles, tendons, and ligaments that are less likely to give way under stress and helps reduce the risk of

Benefits of these yoga-inspired workouts:

- Yoga is time-tested over 5,000 years to be safe, effective, and inspiring.
- These workouts do not require any high-priced trainers or expensive memberships. The biggest investment is your time and your dedication, and I know you are already motivated to succeed!
- These workouts are designed for everybody, whether you are experienced with training and want to try the advanced exercises or are just beginning to create workouts for yourself.
- The book is designed to stave off boredom by giving six weeks of options and three levels to achieve. The Beginner-level workouts are

also shorter in duration, so if you are crunched for time one day, there are *no excuses* to skip your workouts.

The results you can expect from *Body Sculpting with Yoga* are more vast than if you were to stick to just one type of workout, because with these workouts you get the benefits of the cross-training philosophy. By mixing up the moves, continually moving, and adding resistance and creative activities, you can expect:

- Toned legs and thighs
- Chiseled arms
- Buns of steel
- No more saggy triceps
- Tighter abdominals
- Stronger back
- Overall muscle definition
- Reduction of visible cellulite
- Better body symmetry
- Fewer injuries
- More flexibility overall
- Increased concentration
- Improved focus
- Mental toughness
- Increased energy
- Faster recovery
- Better joint stability
- Reduced joint pain
- Better bone density
- Increased confidence
- Fat loss
- Increased functionality of all organs
- Improved breathing patterns
- Reduced stress
- Better sleep

Take Your Workout Wherever You Go

This workout is convenient and simple. It can go anywhere with you and requires little to no extra equipment. When you are at home and can rock through the training, try adding equipment and props for an extra challenge (see pages 24-25 for a list of equipment). If you are traveling or on vacation, follow the Beginner level with no extra equipment. Just do multiple sets, and you'll never miss a day of training!

Pairing my long-time love of weightlifting with my innate devotion and passion for yoga, the workouts in this book are a perfect progression and blend of exercises to share with everyone. This type of training gives you the best of both worlds. The yoga aspects will enhance your posture, elongate your muscles for maximum range of motion, and teach you the importance of breathing, flexibility, and focus. All of these yoga benefits—together with the increased strength and muscle mass of weight training, improved bone density from using resistance, and quick bursts of aerobic activity—come together to create the best, most complete workout.

The benefits of this hybrid yoga workout are exciting and real. By combining the compelling benefits of yoga and weight training, these workouts will offer some amazing results in the way you look and feel.

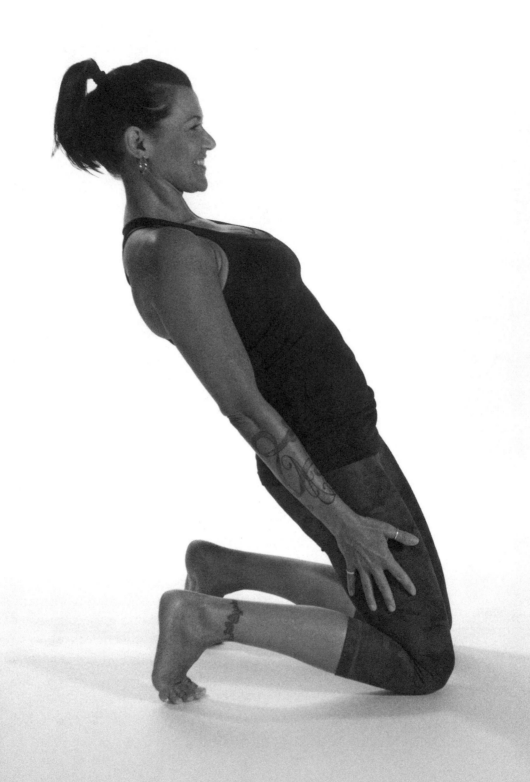

Nutrition Tips

3

Now that you know about all of the amazing results you can achieve by following these workouts, let's talk about another crucial component in reaching your fitness goals—nutrition.

In addition to adding regular yoga and weight training with the *Body Sculpting with Yoga* workouts, you will also need to learn the importance of eating the right way for YOU. After all, you are only as good as the nutrients you put into your body.

About five years ago, I was in tremendous pain throughout my entire body. Every joint movement was agonizing. I was healthy, I worked out, did not drink, did not smoke, was a vegetarian since the age of 10, and was careful about what I put into my body. Despite my healthy lifestyle, something was clearly not right. I felt like a science experiment, going from doctor to doctor and undergoing test after test, all to no avail.

After months of this uncertainty, I was finally diagnosed with rheumatoid arthritis. I could not believe what I was hearing—that is a death sentence for a yoga teacher. I felt

puzzled, frustrated, and confused.

One morning, I was teaching yoga to one of my elite MLB players. While waiting for him, I started chatting with his cook. She said to me, "Ya know, Gwen, everything can be healed by your diet!" This statement intrigued me, but also made me angry because I thought I *was* eating right.

Soon after, I learned about a cleanse with the philosophy of elimination, restoration, and rejuvenation. It sounded good, but I had done cleanses before and knew that they could sometimes be dangerous to your health, so I approached this new cleanse carefully. This approach seemed different. It was about eliminating all potential allergens for 21 days and making your body's Ph more alkaline and less acidic, because an acidic body feeds disease and illness.

The basis of this cleanse was not starvation. In this program, you are actually "allowed" to eat, and eat *smart*. So I gave it a shot.

By day four, I was pain-free in my joints for the first time in three years! I was motivated, inspired, and excited—I felt great!

The key to this cleanse is to systematically remove specific foods from your diet, and then add them back in one at a time so that you can actually see how your body responds. The end goal is to identify any possible allergens in your foods that may be wreaking havoc on your body, and then eliminating these allergens so that your body can function better.

I really encourage you to try this cleanse technique prior to rebuilding your body and committing to a healthier, stronger, more sculpted you. Your body will respond to the workouts better and you will see results faster.

My identified allergen was soy. While on the cleanse, I met with a very gifted doctor. He started talking to me about soy and how

bad it is for you, and suggested I read the book *The Whole Soy Story*. I did and my mind was spinning. I have been a vegetarian since age 10 and ate tofu and soy products regularly in the pursuit of finding the right amount of protein for my body. I knew by the end of this astoundingly informative book that soy was the culprit. It was in *everything*. I finally cleaned it all out of my diet and now after more than three years, I do not have any joint pain at all and my migraines have decreased significantly.

The 10 Adverse Effects of Unfermented Soy on Your Body

1. Reduces assimilation of calcium, magnesium, copper, iron, and zinc.

2. Interferes with protein digestion and may cause pancreatic disorders.

3. In test animals, trypsin inhibitors in soy caused stunted growth.

4. Increases potent agents that block your synthesis of thyroid hormones and can cause hypothyroidism and thyroid cancer. In infants, consumption of soy formula has been linked with autoimmune thyroid disease.

5. Contains plant compounds resembling human estrogen, which can block your normal estrogen and disrupt endocrine function, cause infertility, and increase your risk for breast cancer.

6. Soy has a clot-promoting substance that causes your red blood cells to clump, making them unable to properly absorb and distribute oxygen to your tissues.

7. Soy foods increase your body's vitamin D requirement, which is why companies add synthetic vitamin D to soymilk.

8. Soy contains a compound resembling vitamin B12 that cannot be used by your body, so soy foods can actually contribute to B12 deficiency, especially among vegans.

9. MSG, a potent neurotoxin, is formed during soy food processing, and additional MSG is often added to mask soy's unpleasant taste.

10. Soy foods contain high levels of aluminum, which is toxic to your nervous system and kidneys, as well as manganese, which wreaks havoc on babies' immature metabolic systems.

Clean Eating Guide

Whenever I need a nutritional boost, I follow these basic
guidelines for three to four days, two or three times a year:

Good Foods	Foods to Eliminate
Fruits: Whole and unsweetened frozen	Oranges, orange juice, grapefruit, strawberries, grapes, bananas
Dairy substitutes: Rice, oat, and nut milks	Milk, cheese, cottage cheese, cream, yogurt, butter, ice cream, non-dairy creamer
Non-gluten grains: Brown rice, millet, quinoa, amaranth, buckwheat	Wheat, corn, barley, spelt, kamut, rye, couscous, oats
Animal protein: Cold water fish, wild game, lean lamb, duck, chicken, turkey	Raw fish, pork, beef, veal, sausage, deli meats, canned meats, hot dogs, shellfish, eggs
Vegetable protein: Split peas, lentils, and legumes	Soybean products, peanuts, peanut butter, pistachios, macadamia nuts
Nuts and seeds: Sesame seeds, pumpkin seeds, sunflower seeds, hazelnuts, pecans, almonds, cashews, walnuts	Corn, creamed vegetables, tomatoes, potatoes, eggplants, peppers
Vegetables: Fresh and raw, steamed, sautéed, juiced, roasted	Butter, margarine, shortening, processed oils, salad dressings, mayonnaise, spreads
Oils: Cold-pressed olive, flax, safflower, sesame, almond, sunflower, canola, pumpkin, walnut	Alcohol, coffee, caffeinated beverages, soda, soft drinks
Drinks: Filtered or distilled water, green tea, herbal tea, seltzer, yerba mate	Refined sugar, white or brown sugars, honey, maple syrup, high-fructose corn syrup, evaporated cane juice
Sweeteners: Brown rice syrup, agave, stevia	
Condiments: Vinegar, all spices, sea salt, pepper, basil, carob, cinnamon, cumin, dill, garlic, ginger, mustard, oregano, parsley, rosemary, turmeric, thyme	Chocolate, ketchup, relish, chutney, soy sauce, barbecue sauce, teriyaki sauce, and other similar sauces

Timing Your Meals

In addition to my profound experience and belief in clean eating and living, I also believe in being diligent about letting your body recover each day. If you want your body to focus on its ability to get stronger, leaner, and more fit, you have to relieve it of the duties of detoxing and complicated digestion processes so your results from these workouts will be apparent even sooner. In order to give your body this time to recover, it's important to look at *when* you eat and *what* you eat at certain times throughout the day. I personally feel best when I stop eating in the evening at 7 PM and do not eat again in the morning until 9 or even 10 AM. I feel I am giving my digestive system the break it needs to thrive and reboot. Play around with these hours. The most important point is to stop bingeing on snacks and treats in the evening right before bed, which only bombards your body when it needs to rest and rejuvenate, not digest.

Food Combining

Another important part of healthy nutrition is food combining. Improper food combining is one of the primary factors that cause flatulence, heartburn, and upset stomach. What's worse, poor digestion can also contribute to malnutrition, even if you think you're eating a decent diet.

The basic rules of food combining include:

- Do not eat proteins and starches together. Your body requires an acid base to digest proteins and an alkaline base to digest starches. Proteins and starches combine well with green, leafy vegetables and non-starchy vegetables, but they do not combine well with each other.
- Generally, fruits should be eaten alone or with other fruits. If fruits seem too sweet, then eat a handful of nuts (80 percent fruit, 20 percent nuts). Fruits digest so quickly that by the time they reach your stomach, they are already partially digested. If they are combined with other foods, they will rot and ferment.
- Eat only four to six different fruits or vegetables at one meal.
- Fats and oils combine with everything (except fruits) but should be used in limited amounts. While they won't inhibit digestion, they will slow it down.
- Wait the following lengths of time between meals that don't combine:
  - o Two hours after eating fruit
  - o Three hours after eating starches
  - o Four hours after eating proteins

The When and What of Eating

According to nutritional expert Dr. Wayne Pickering (www.wayne-pickering.com), the amount and sequencing of the foods you eat can also make a difference. He recommends the following eating schedule:

- **Morning meal:** The least concentrated foods, in the greatest amount. Ideal food choice: fruits.
- **Middle of the day:** More complex foods, but in a smaller amount than your first meal. Ideal food choice: starchy carbs.
- **Evening:** The most concentrated foods, but in the least abundant amount. Ideal food choice: protein.

Sample Meal Plan

BREAKFAST

Breakfast Smoothie

4 cups watermelon, cantaloupe, and honeydew melon
1 cup apple juice
1 cup ice cubes

Place all ingredients in a blender and blend until smooth.

Fruit Salad

10-15 large strawberries, rinsed and quartered
2 cups blueberrles
2 cups pineapple chunks
2 cups watermelon cubes
2 cups melon
2 kiwis
1 peach
1 pear
1 mango

Combine all ingredients.

LUNCH

Vegetable Soup

3 tablespoons olive oil
1 large onion
1 leek
3 carrots
2 stalks celery
4 garlic cloves, pressed
1½ cups fresh green beans, trimmed
6 cups organic vegetable broth
1 bay leaf
¼ teaspoon thyme
1 cup peas
3 small zucchini, diced
1 (15-ounce) can cannellini beans, rinsed and drained

In a large soup pot, heat olive oil over medium heat. Add onion and leek and sauté for 4 minutes. Add carrots, celery, and garlic and cook over medium heat for another 5 minutes. Add green beans and cook 5 more minutes.

Add broth, bay leaf, and thyme and stir well. Bring to a boil, reduce heat, and cover; let simmer for 20 minutes.

Add peas and simmer 10 more minutes. Stir in zucchini, peas, and cannellini beans and simmer for 10 minutes. Remove bay leaf and serve.

Tuna Salad

1 can organic white tuna
2 tablespoons vinegar
1 tablespoons olive oil
Dash of lemon juice
3 tablespoons shelled unsalted raw sunflower seeds
1 bunch kale
Salt, pepper, and dill, to taste
Mix tuna, vinegar, oil, salt, pepper, lemon, dill, and sunflower seeds. Serve on a bed of fresh kale, seasoned to taste, with a side of quinoa.

DINNER

Salmon with Glaze

¾ cup dry white wine
¼ cup coconut milk
1 tablespoon butter

2 tablespoons Old Bay seasoning
2 pounds salmon fillets
1/3 cup spicy brown mustard
¼ cup agave syrup

Preheat oven to 375°F. Combine wine, coconut milk, butter, and Old Bay seasoning in a small saucepan; bring to a boil and simmer for 5 minutes. Place fish in a baking dish, and pour the wine-coconut milk-butter sauce over the fish. Bake for 5 minutes. Meanwhile, combine mustard and agave in a bowl. Remove fish from oven and change heat to broil. Spread mustard-agave mixture over the fish, place under broiler, and broil until top is bubbly, approximately 3 to 5 minutes. Serve with steamed green beans mixed with almonds.

Spicy Red Beans and Rice

3 tablespoons olive oil
1 medium onion, chopped
3 garlic cloves, minced
1 stalk celery, chopped
1½ teaspoons thyme
½ teaspoon cayenne pepper
3 cups vegetable broth
1½ cups brown rice
½ teaspoon seasoned salt
1 (16-ounce) can kidney beans, rinsed and drained

Heat oil in large pot over medium heat. Add onion, garlic, celery, thyme, and cayenne and sauté until tender, about 10 minutes. Stir in broth, rice, and seasoned salt. Bring to a boil, cover, reduce heat, and simmer for 20 minutes or until rice is tender. Add beans, stir, and heat for a few minutes. Serve with tossed salad.

Food No-No's

- Soda
- White flour and white sugar
- Alcohol (in excess)
- Salt (in excess)
- Soy
- Artificial colors and artificial flavors

Remember, you are only as good as the nutrients you put into your body.

Daily Life Skills

Your body needs more than conscious eating and regular exercise. Below are six daily practices for better overall health. Add one idea each week as you begin a new week of workouts. By the end of the six weeks you will:

- See a new body emerge
- Follow a new way of eating
- See allergies reduced
- Feel cleaner and clearer

Week one: Start a morning meditation. When your alarm goes off in the morning, stop, inhale and exhale deeply 10 times with your eyes closed, then get up and get ready for your day. Deep breathing eases stress, oxygenates and cleanses the body, and starts your day on the right foot.

Week two: Try dry skin brushing, which opens up the pores, tightens skin, and promotes cell renewal and blood flow. Your skin should be dry, so the ideal time is in the shower before you turn on the water (don't get the brush wet). Brush toward the heart, making long sweeps. Start at your feet, moving up the legs on both sides, then work from the arms toward your chest. On your stomach, direct the brush counterclockwise. Don't brush too hard; your skin should be stimulated and invigorated but not irritated or red. Use a brush with natural bristles that are somewhat stiff, though not too hard.

Week three: Drink more water. My rule of thumb for water is to drink half my body weight in ounces each day. Water is one of the best tools for weight loss and a healthier, more efficient body. It replaces high-calorie drinks like soda and juice and is also a great appetite suppressant.

Being dehydrated can drain your energy and make you feel tired. If you're thirsty, you're already dehydrated, and this can lead to fatigue, muscle weakness, dizziness, and headaches. Drinking a healthy amount of water is also good for the skin and helps the body to digest food properly and flush out toxins and waste products.

Week four: Get rest. Commit to allowing yourself the time to get at least seven hours of sleep per night. It may take some planning, but it is well worth it. Sleep deprivation can cause weight gain by altering hormone levels and affecting the way the body processes and stores carbohydrates, and has also been linked to hypertension, increased stress hormones, and irregular heartbeat.

Week five: Massage. You do not have to spend extravagant amounts of money getting a massage—all you have to do is take some time after your shower to firmly and thoroughly massage a natural cream or oil into your body (I use coconut oil or sesame oil). If you are fortunate enough to be able to afford professional massages, four to 12 per year is recommended. Or, consider a trade with a friend.

Week six: Keep a journal. Writing helps organize your thoughts, and journaling takes it to a new level. It can help you form and organize goals, and process which are most important to you. People tend to be more truthful with themselves when journaling and often feelings can surface more openly in a setting that is calm and allows you to sort through your emotions more rationally. Journaling is also a great venue to write down significant experiences in your life and organize your feelings toward them.

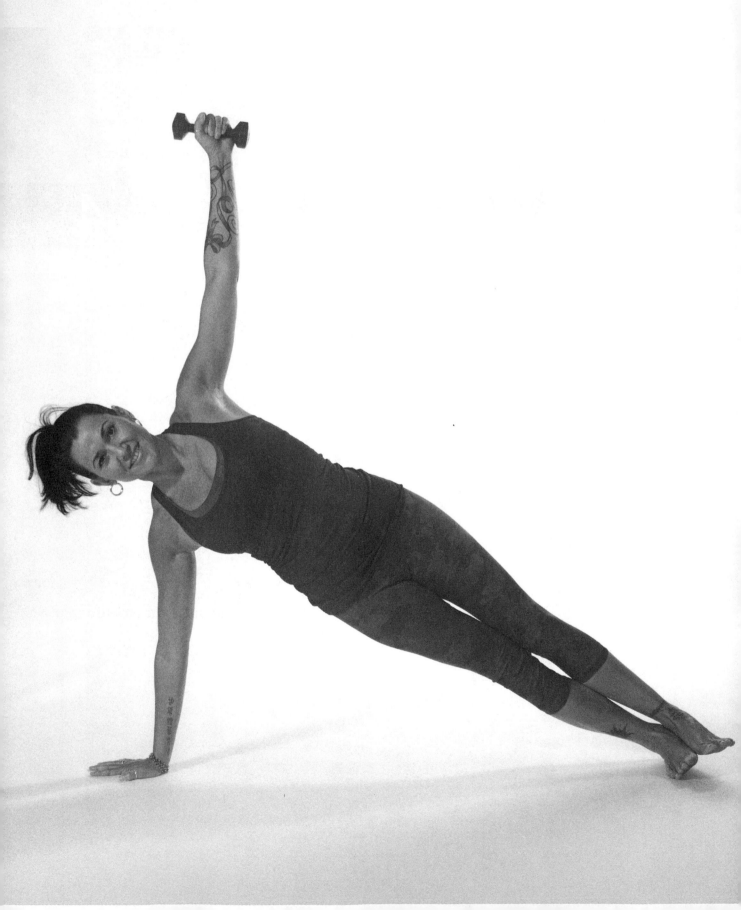

About the **Workouts**

4

Now that you are fully motivated and have more complete guidance on your nutritional needs, let's get started! It's time to map out your workout space, clothing, and equipment to maximize your results and track your progress.

Prepping for Your Workout

All you need to get started are a few basic items:

- **Mat:** A yoga mat that has some cushion to protect your joints and some tack to avoid slipping.
- **Proper clothing:** Proper clothing includes loose-fitting pants that allow you to do deep moves, but are not so loose that the fabric will get in your way. When choosing shirts, a tight fitting tank top usually works well.
- **Timer:** To help with some of the moves that are based on time rather than reps.

What to Wear

Some women love to wear short shorts or loose shorts when working out, but I would not recommend wearing these for the yoga-inspired workouts in this book. You want to feel confident that you're totally covered when doing all of the movements. When you're bending or twisting, the last thing you want to think about is whether someone can see something they should not be seeing, or become distracted because you have to frequently adjust the position of your shorts to be properly covered.

The best option is to choose fitted, cropped, or full-length leggings. You will be fully covered, and the material will also absorb sweat.

T-shirts and loose tank tops are usually not the best choice for working out or for doing yoga because they will just end up falling over your head every time you come into a compromising position. Instead, try long, fitted tanks that will stay put and keep you covered even if you twist, bend backward, or flip upside down. Also, you will not have sleeves to hinder a deep twist or difficult movement.

Choosing what to wear on your feet can also be difficult because it is specific to how you are most comfortable. I choose to work out barefoot, so my yoga moves move seamlessly to my workout moves. If you prefer to wear shoes, choose a lightweight, very pliable sneaker and moisture-wicking socks.

For Intermediate and Advanced workouts, you can also add the following equipment for a tougher challenge:

Wrist and ankle weights

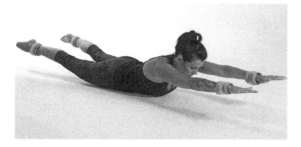

Weight vest

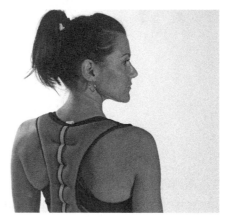

Light dumbbells

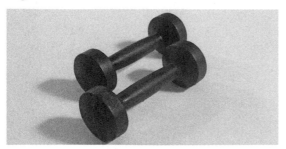

Light kettlebells

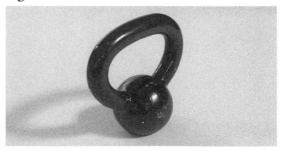

(*The equipment on page 24 will add resistance and weight to your moves, which helps to build sleek, long muscle while increasing your cardio output.*)

Sandbag: Strategically hold the sand bag or position it on your body so that you can sink deeper into a move.

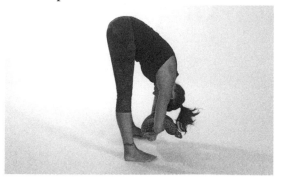

Medicine ball: Adds a different resistance and also helps build muscle and raises the heart rate.

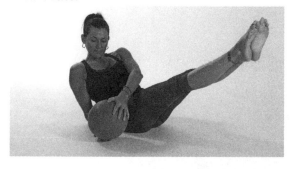

Isometric bands: Adds resistance to an exercise without adding additional weights.

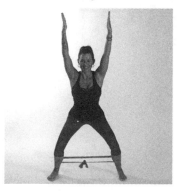

How to Follow the Workouts

This book is designed to be user-friendly and is customizable to *your* body and *your* fitness goals. The workouts are arranged into three levels—Beginner, Intermediate, and Advanced—with six weeks of workouts for each level. You will work out four days each week (we recommend Monday, Wednesday, Friday, and Saturday) and for each day you will find clear directions on when and how to perform the workouts. Pick your level of fitness and follow the guide. The duration of the workouts is completely determined by you and should be based on the goals you have set for yourself. The workouts are set up as a continuous flow, and at the end of the flow (depending on your energy level and time constraints) you will repeat the flow one to three more times.

As you become more adept at the workouts, you can choose to add additional weights to increase resistance, build more muscle, and increase your heart rate. You can start by adding ½- to 1-pound wrist and/or ankle weights. Later on, you may also want to add a 10- to 15-pound weighted vest.

The workouts are designed for each exercise to move seamlessly into the next in a smooth, yoga-inspired way. You may want to review the moves first and visualize how your body will move through the poses before you start. A great idea is to prop the book up in front of you to avoid having to walk back and forth to note the next move, and make sure to set up your equipment for each workout before you begin so that you can keep the flow constant.

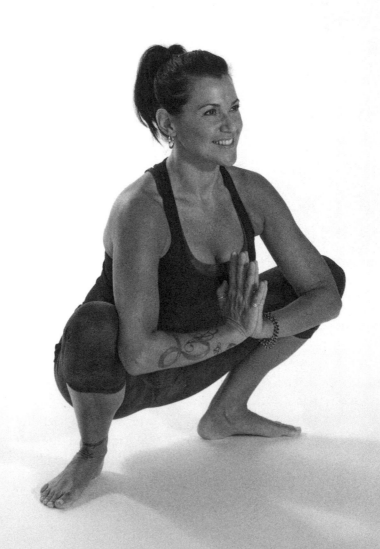

Setting Your
Fitness Goals

5

You've already made the decision to change your life by getting your body in shape. You have learned about the workouts and exercises you will be following, gained some helpful nutritional guidance, and now you're eager to get started!

Before you dive into the workouts, take some time to sit down and set your fitness goals; you can greatly increase the likelihood of reaching your expectations. You would never decide to build a house, meet the builder, and just throw a bunch of nails, wood, and sheetrock at him and say, "Build it!" No way! Instead, you take months to carefully plan and create a set of directives to build the house you want. It is the same concept with your fitness goals.

All too frequently people just go about their days wishing and hoping without taking action. Now, it is time to take action, and actually design the life you have been dreaming.

First, you need to have a vision for what you want your fitness goals to be. In any sport, athletes visualize scoring that winning goal or throwing that perfect pass. Goals give you long-term vision and short-term motivation. In goal-setting, we visualize exactly what we want our life to look like in the years to come. From that vision, we can create the life that we are truly meant to be living. We all lead by example, so when you have goals set for yourself in your life, you will also inspire others to want to do the same. Goal-setting is a very powerful way of motivating people, including you! Let's get started...

"Good is the enemy of great." —Jim Collins

Focusing Your Goals

Below is a list of questions you can ask yourself to help you uncover your fitness goals and start paving the way to making them a reality. You may want to print these out and carry them with you so that you can add to your goal-setting every day!

Ask yourself these questions:

- Are you living your dreams?
- Are you happy every day?
- What would you be doing if you knew you could not fail?
- Is every day full of possibility?
- Are you happy with your body?
- Are you setting a healthy example for the people around you?

If the answer to any of these is "no," then now is the perfect time for you to dig in and be the change you wish to see in your life!

"All that we are is the result of what we have thought."
—Buddha

COMMON THINKING	NEW THINKING
"It will be difficult."	"Anything is possible."
"It will take a long time."	"I cannot fail when I plan and trust in myself."
"I do not deserve it."	"There is only now—I will live fully in the present."
"It is not my nature."	"Everyone deserves the chance to achieve their dreams."
"I cannot afford it."	"If I can conceive of it, my passion and abilities will make it happen."
"No one will help me."	"I am committed to being an example of healthy living to all my loved ones."
"I am not strong enough."	"I live in the body that makes me happy."
"I am not smart enough."	"I am fit and feel great every day."
"I am too busy."	
"I am too scared."	

In order to create your ideal body and reach your fitness goals in the body you always wanted, you need to start with a clear vision.

- Close your eyes.
- Where do you see yourself in 10 years?

Be as specific as possible, down to the color of the sheets that you sleep on!

Open your eyes now, grab a pen and paper and begin your brainstorm. Write as much as you possibly can about what you *truly* want in your life, in terms of your fitness and the body you always wanted, as if nothing could stop you. You might not know but once you start putting your thoughts to paper, ideas will come out that will surprise you. Get everything out on paper first, we will hone in on what is important later. If you think that you want it for yourself, write it down. Thing BIG! Write down lofty goals. Get crazy. If you see yourself as the next top fitness model, or as a professional athlete, or walking on the beach this year confident and strong, write it down. This is for you—it is personal, so be honest with yourself.

Write what you are good at in health and in fitness; do not leave anything out. Now, to know what your gifts are, ask three people in your life the following questions and write down all the answers. I guarantee you will be inspired and humbled, and will feel ready to design the body and life you want.

- What are my key strengths?
- What is most unique about me?
- When the goal gets tough, do I quit?
- Could I be an inspiration to others?
- Could you tell me something about myself that I do not already know?
- When am I most powerful?
- In what situation am I least powerful?
- When am I most inspired?
- If you could wish one thing for me in this next year, what would it be?

After the interviews:

- Do you see patterns and trends in the responses?
- What responses stand out and why?
- Write out five of your past health and fitness successes and figure out how to duplicate them.

- Write out five failures and learn from them.
- Write out any incompletions and finish them or move on to a new goal.

Now that you have your vision brainstormed, you are ready to start breaking it down so that you can focus on the most important health and fitness goals.

Goals are set on a number of different levels. First you create your "big picture" of what you want and decide what large-scale goals you want to achieve; in this case, what you want your body and your health to look like. Second, you break these down into the smaller targets that you must hit so you can reach your goals; for example, what workouts you will do on what days and how you will alter your eating patterns and surroundings to support that goal. Finally, once you have your plan, you put your plan into action and get ready to achieve what you set out to.

Benefits of Setting Goals

- Goal-setting helps you decide what is important for you to achieve in your life.
- It sets apart what is important from what is irrelevant or distracting.
- It motivates you.
- It builds your self-confidence.

POST YOUR GOALS! Write them down and paste them up around your home as gentle reminders of what you are working toward. You can do anything that you set your mind to!

"Far better is it to dare mighty things, to win glorious triumphs, even though checkered by failure, than to take rank with those poor spires who neither enjoy much nor suffer much because they live in the gray twilight that knows not victory or defeat."

—Theodore Roosevelt

Tips for Staying on Track

- Accept *total* responsibility for everything that happens in your life.
- Revisit your goals often.
- Revise goals if necessary.
- Find a goal buddy and help each other to stay on track.
- Share your goals with people you trust so that they can help motivate you.
- Create visual reminders of your goals (such as a vision board).
- If you get off track, realize it…then forgive and restart.
- Move forward constantly; take action every day.

Tips for Writing Powerful Goals

- Always write goals in the first person and present tense, as though they already have been achieved.
- Use clear and specific words that demonstrate commitment.
- The mind likes a specific number; include them in your goals.
- Allow yourself to see pictures of your life as you dream.
- Always write goals in the affirmative.
- Always include a timeline with each goal.
- Look ahead to the future if you need clarity.

"I can accept failure, everyone fails at something. But I can't accept not trying"

—Michael Jordan

Streaming Thought: What is your 10-year vision?

Personal:_____

_____

_____

_____

Health:_____

_____

_____

_____

Fitness:_____

_____

_____

_____

Streaming Thought: What is your five-year vision?

Personal: _____

_____

_____

_____

Health:_____

_____

_____

_____

Fitness:_____

_____

_____

_____

Streaming Thought: What is your one-year vision?

Personal: _____

_____

_____

_____

Health: _____

_____

_____

_____

Fitness: _____

_____

_____

_____

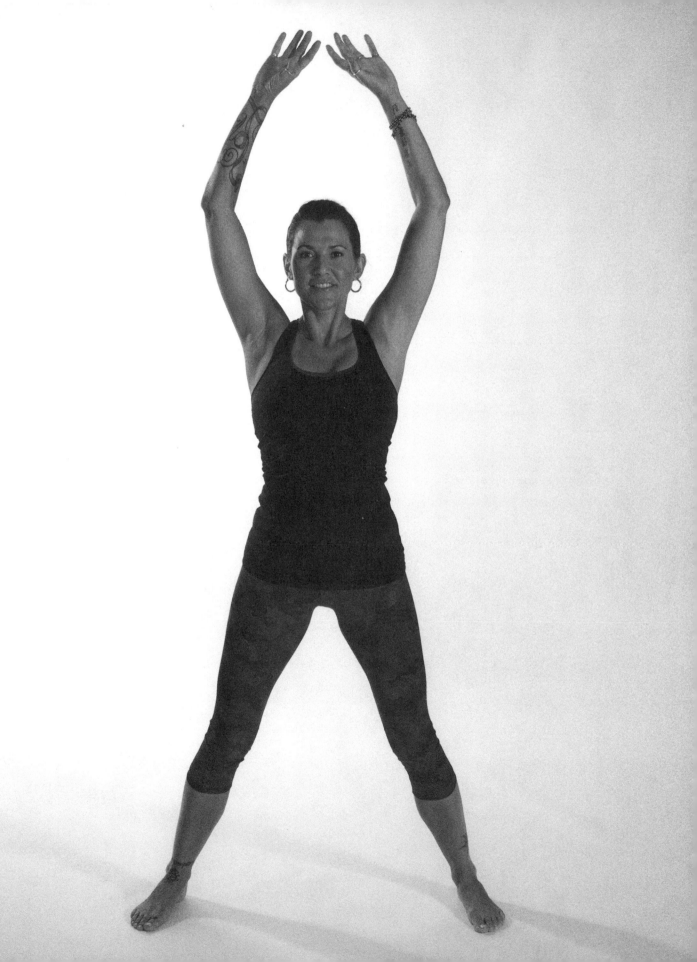

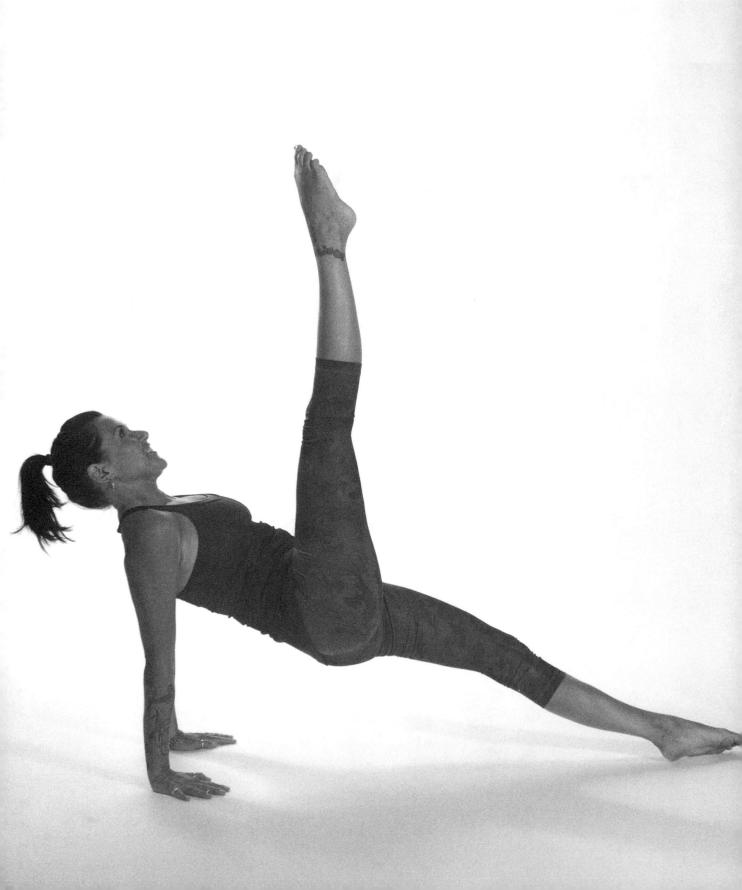

Part II:
The Body Sculpting with Yoga Workout

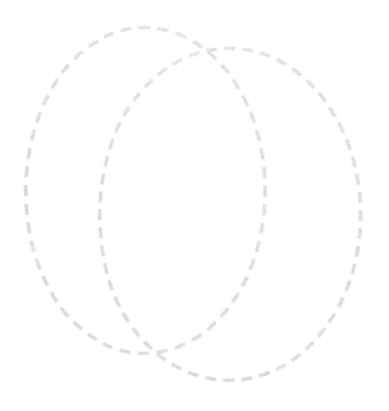

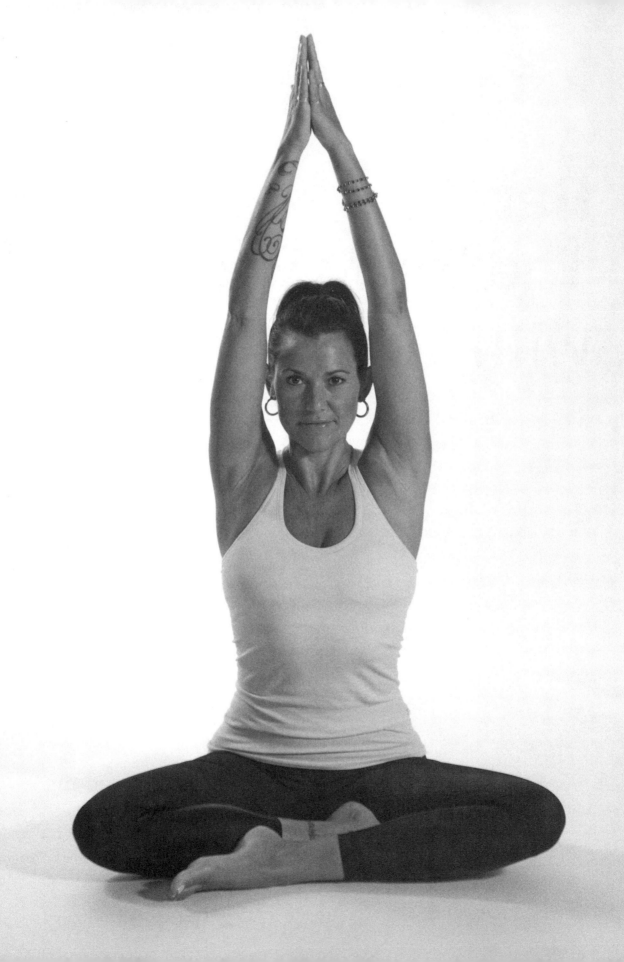

Warm-Ups and Cool-Downs

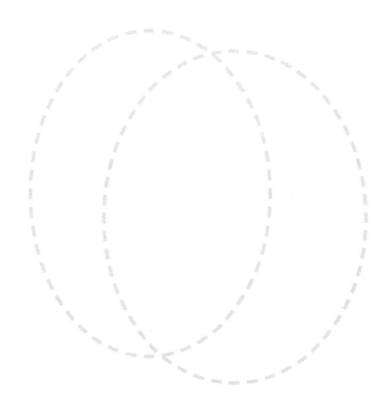

Pre-Workout: Assessment Poses

Starting each workout with these assessment moves will help you to identify any imbalances before they become injuries. I find that starting with the same moves each time gives your body a clear message as to what is coming and helps you to prepare for your workout, both physically and mentally. Do not skip these warm-ups—your body will love you for it.

Why I recommend warming up:

- Increases blood flow to the muscles, joints, and connective tissue

- Increases oxygenation

- Gives you an opportunity to tune in and identify any tight places or pain

- Gives you an opportunity to mentally prepare for your workout

Perform each of the warm-up moves on pages 38-39 before every workout.

Twist

Sitting cross-legged in a comfortable position with a tall back, position your arms at a 90-degree angle from the body and twist for two minutes. Sync your breathing with the movement and start to become aware of which way it is easiest for you to twist and which way you have more resistance so you can improve and fix that imbalance later. After two minutes, take a deep breath and a full exhale.

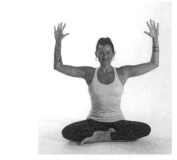

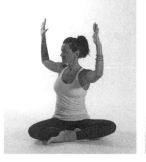

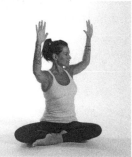

Arm Ups

Sitting in cross-legged position in a comfortable position, inhale and bring the arms up overhead and exhale bringing the arms down. When the arms go up, the palms should be face up and when the arms go down, the palms should be face down. Do this for two minutes; it will challenge the shoulder muscles and you will feel the instant warmth in the shoulder joint.

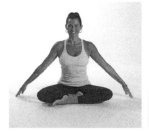

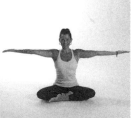

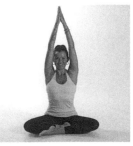

Opposite Arm, Opposite Leg

Lying down on your back, take a full body stretch and reach out your arms and legs as far as possible. (This will probably induce a yawn, which I call the "full body yawn".) Press your lower back into the floor and proceed to touch the opposite arm to the opposite leg, keeping your head relaxed on the floor. After time, your fingertips will touch the tips of your toes; this indicates a nice, open set of hamstrings. While you are performing this warm-up move, become aware of which hamstring is tighter and which one feels great so you can become better aware of your imbalances. Do this for two minutes. If you can, exhale when the arms and legs go up and inhale when they lower.

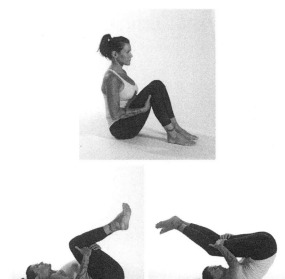

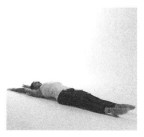
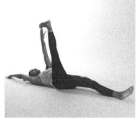

Rock and Rolls

While lying on your back, draw your knees into your chest and wrap your arms behind your thighs to avoid over-flexing the knee with the upper body strength. Rock and roll vigorously for a full minute (just like you did when as a kid). This move will bring a smile to your face and will stimulate your spine and all the nerves, increase blood flow, and gently help align your vertebra.

Wipers

While lying on your back, bend the knees into the chest and place a soft yoga block or a rolled up towel between your inner thighs. Extend your arms out directly from your shoulders with palms facing down for support. Drop your knees all the way over, from one side to the other. This will warm up your abdominals and lower back. Do this for two minutes.

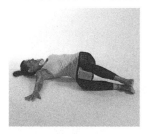
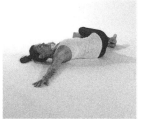
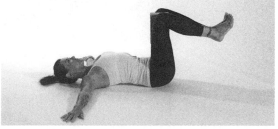

Post-Workout: Long Deep Holds

These post-workout movements will increase flexibility, train your mind, and hone your focus. Choose three post-workout movements to perform after each workout. Mix them up each day to keep your workout interesting and to target different areas of the body.

Plow

Plow is a great pose to do after a vigorous workout. It will release stress from the upper body, neck, and shoulders. It is a gentle inversion, so it also helps the body to flush out toxins and changes your perspective. Do this pose for three to five minutes while breathing deeply and consistently.

Lying on your back, draw your knees into your chest and gently press your legs up over your body and head. Some people will be able to touch their toes to the floor above their head. If your toes touch, snuggle your shoulders under and try to interlace your fingers, extending your arms. If your toes do not touch the floor, then bend your elbows and place your hands flat on your back to support yourself.

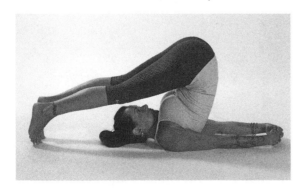

Open Chest Stretch

This is a favorite of mine and I believe every person in the world can benefit from this pose on the physio-ball. It will open the chest; decompress the spine; clear the lungs; increase deep respirations; and stretch the biceps, quads, and hip flexors. It also reverses the effects of poor posture and enables the organs to function better.

While sitting on the physio-ball, walk your feet forward until you are lying on the ball (play around with the positioning of the ball to where you feel the best support and stretch). Let your arms hang out to the side and relax your head back. Hold this position for three to 10 minutes.

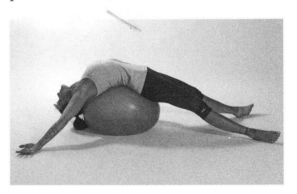

Forward Bend

This pose is most effective when done against a wall. The wall will support you so you do not have to constantly worry about your balance, and leaning against the wall allows the hamstrings to open more and become more flexible. Do this pose for one to three minutes; it will really test your will. Be careful when coming out of the pose— bend the knees and drop down to a seated position; *do not* stand as you will likely get dizzy.

Stand facing a wall with your toes about 8 to 10 inches from the wall. Your feet should be parallel and hips width apart. Bend your knees deeply and start to fold forward so your chest and belly rest against your thighs. When you fold over, be careful not to bump your head on the wall. Place your hands on the floor for better stability, then lean the back of your head and back completely against the wall. As you sink in and improve on this stretch you will be able to straighten your legs more and more until they are totally straight and most of your back touches the wall. Inhale and exhale, lean, and let gravity take you down. If your heels come off the floor while you are doing this, adjust the distance of your feet to the wall until they are flat. If only the back of your head touches the wall because your hamstrings are tight, bend your knees more so your back is against the wall. Hold and breathe.

hands and turn the thigh out so the right knee does not point straight ahead, but points to about 1 or 2 o'clock. Slide the left leg straight back as far as you can. You may rest on your forearms or all the way down to your chest. It is important that your hips are square and you are not resting on your right hip and that you do not feel knee pain in this position. Hold, then repeat on the other side.

If you are a beginner and you cannot sink in deeply, or if you have knee problems, place a block under the bent knee hip for support.

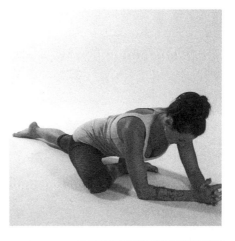

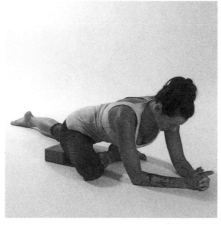

Pigeon

This pose is the kingpin for opening sore, tight glutes and for releasing pressure on the sciatic nerve. Do this pose for three to five minutes on each leg; focus on relaxing and releasing the belly and neck while sinking in.

Starting on your hands and knees, slide the right knee forward between your

Frog

A staple in my regimen, this pose opens the groin and inner thighs, elongating the leg and lessening the impact on the knees. It also builds focus and mental toughness. Hold this pose for three to six minutes; you will learn to love it.

Start on your hands and knees, making sure your hips are directly over your knees. Slowly slide the knees out as far as you can, resting your chest or belly on a block and your head on your hands or the floor. The knees should form a 90-degree angle. Hold.

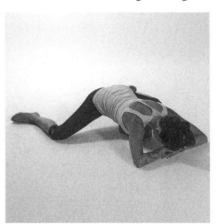

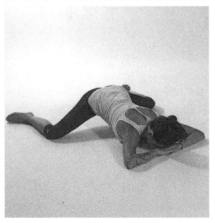

Hero

Hero pose helps to maintain healthy knees. When done properly, it will open the thighs and hip flexors; it also gets a little bit of IT band (the outside of the thigh). In addition, it focuses on the flexibility of the ankle joint by increasing its range of motion. Do this pose for two to five minutes.

Starting on your hands and knees, press your hips back until they can touch your ankles. If you feel knee pain, avoid this pose until your flexibility increases. The idea is to eventually sit straight up with the hips on the heels. Once you can do that, you can sit on a block between your feet. Eventually, you can sit on the floor between your feet. Always keep the bottom of the foot pointing straight up to the sky; *never* have the toes pointing out—it can be very bad for your knees.

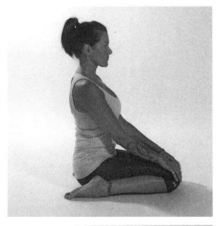

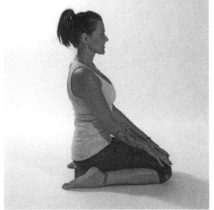

Heavy Legs

You will come to love this pose and will want to do it every day, but remember to mix up your post-workout stretches. This pose is amazing for encouraging lymph drainage and getting rid of that heavy, dead leg feeling you can get when you do tough or long workouts. It is also a great opportunity to do some focused breathing or visualization while you are holding the pose. Do this pose for two to five minutes.

Lie on your back with your feet facing a wall and move toward the wall until your butt is against the wall. Keeping your butt on the ground, swing the legs straight up the wall. If your hamstrings are tight and you cannot straighten your legs without lifting your butt, then ground the hips and bend the knees a little for now.

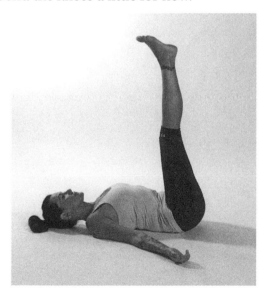

Face Up Shoulder Stretch

This stretch focuses on the front of the shoulders. It opens the rotator cuffs and improves range of motion in the shoulder joints. When done often, it reduces the likelihood of developing bursitis of the shoulder and improves your posture. Hold for two minutes on each side.

Lying on your back, draw your knees into your chest. Drop your knees to the left, bend your right elbow, and place it palm side down under your back. Slowly bring the knees back to center. If you can, gradually drop your knees to the right. Turn your chin over your right shoulder and hold. Your right wrist joint should be covered by your back; otherwise, you will not feel the stretch. Make sure the hand under your back is palm flat, with the fingers extended and spread. Repeat on the other side.

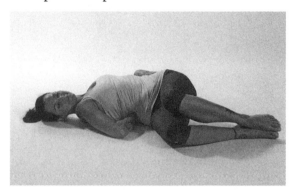

Face Down Shoulder Stretch

This is a great way to wind down after your workout and open the chest, anterior shoulders, and biceps while also adding a spinal twist to the mix. Do this pose for two to four minutes on each side, and be careful to come out slow and controlled.

Lying face down on the floor, extend your right arm out so that the right middle finger is in the eye line and the arm is slightly above the shoulder with flat fingers spread out. Look over your left shoulder, bend the left elbow and bring the left palm under your shoulder like you would for a push-up. Bend the left knee right where it is. Press into the left hand and start to roll over onto your right side with your left foot trying to touch the ground on the floor on the outside of the right leg, with the knee bent and the foot flat. Your left hand supports the pose and presses you deeper into the pose. Eventually the butt will be flat and both knees bent, with both feet flat. Hold, then come out of the pose slowly and repeat on the other side.

Start in a kneeling seated position. Drop your hips to the right of your feet. Situate the right foot so the bottom of the right foot is resting on the top of the left knee. Turn to the right with both hands down on the floor. Extend your spine and continue to twist to the right until you meet resistance. Lower down to your chest and belly. If you cannot reach the floor, place a block or rolled up blanket under your chest and turn your head to the right, trying to rest on your left ear. Your right arm remains bent in a push-up position and your left arm extends over your head, like you were raising your hand. On the inhales, press into your right hand to automatically help you square your chest to the floor and exhale to reach the left arm more. Hold, breathe, come out very slowly, and repeat on the other side.

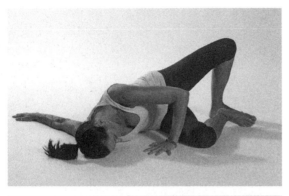

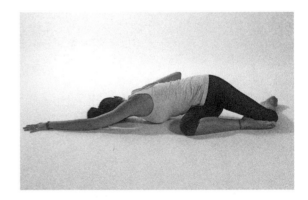

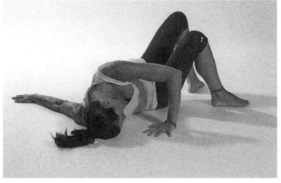

Wheel of Life

The ultimate pose, the Wheel of Life gently aligns and increases rotation of the spine, opens the lats and side body to increase respiration depth, and helps open the IT band and glutes. Hold this pose for three to five minutes on each side. Inhale to deepen the reach and twist of the pose and exhale to sink in.

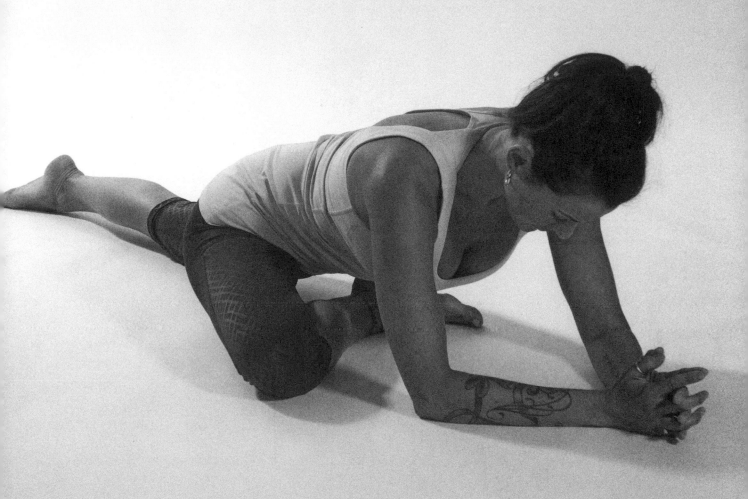

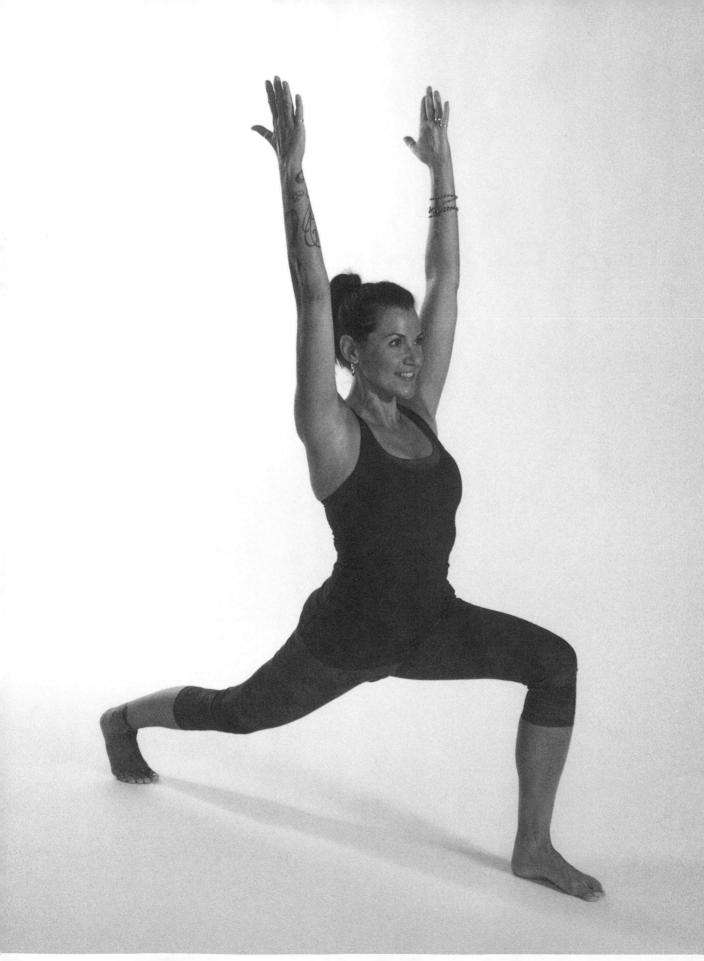

The **Exercises**

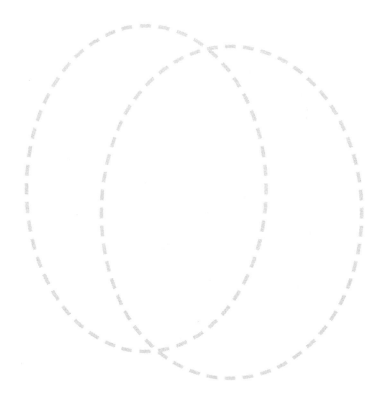

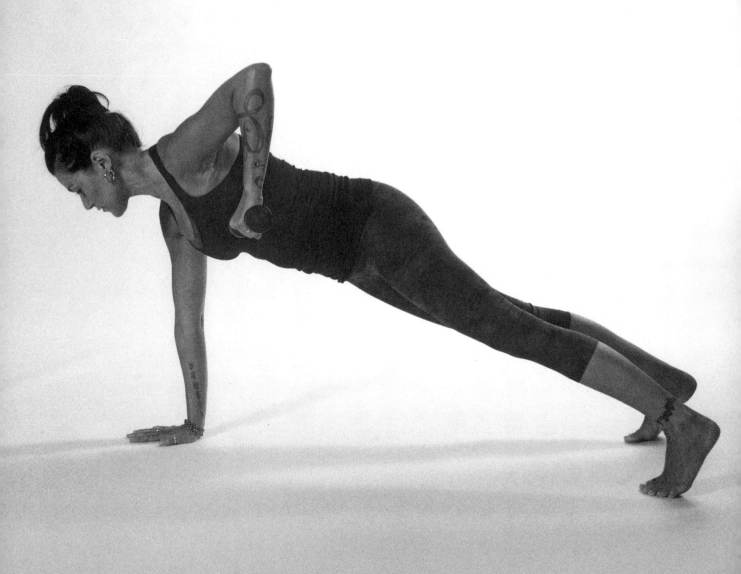

Floor Poses

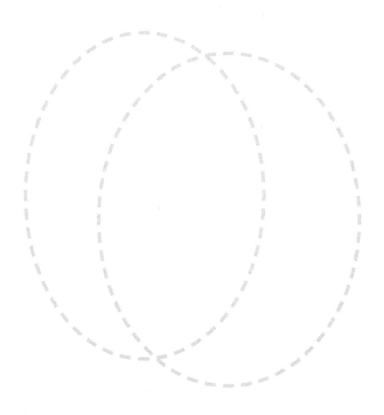

Plank

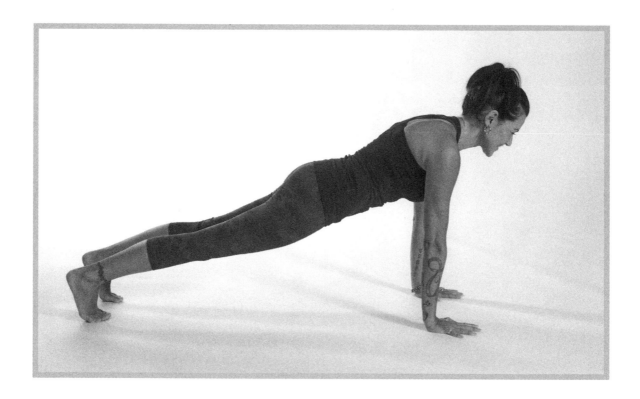

Assume the top position of a push-up. Make sure your wrists are under your elbows, with your elbows under the shoulder joints for the best support. Engage the core. It is important that the hands are flat and the fingers are spread, truly plugging the whole hand into the floor. Make sure to keep equal space between the fingers.

Variations of Plank

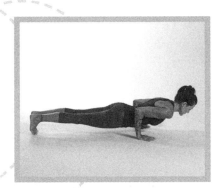

Chateranga

Starting in the same position as Plank, bend the elbows and lower the body to the height of the elbows. Push forward slightly, aiming to have the elbow joints at a 90-degree angle. Hold.

Side to Side Plank

Starting in Plank position, walk two steps to the right and return to center. Walk two steps to the left and return to center.

Plank Scissors

Starting in Plank position, lift the right leg up and down in a scissor motion. Repeat with the left leg.

Raise the Roofs

Starting in Plank position, lift the right leg off the floor and bend the right knee to a 90 degree angle. Flex the right foot and pulse the right leg to the sky. Repeat on the other side.

Knee to Nose

In Plank position, draw your right knee in to kiss the nose and return to Plank. Switch sides and repeat.

Heel Drops

Hold Plank position, keeping the upper body as static as possible. Moving from the waist down, drop the heels from left to right. Keep the core strong and the legs engaged.

Plank Cross-Over

Starting in Plank position, lift the right leg up off the floor, cross it over the left leg, lift, and return to starting position. Repeat on the other side.

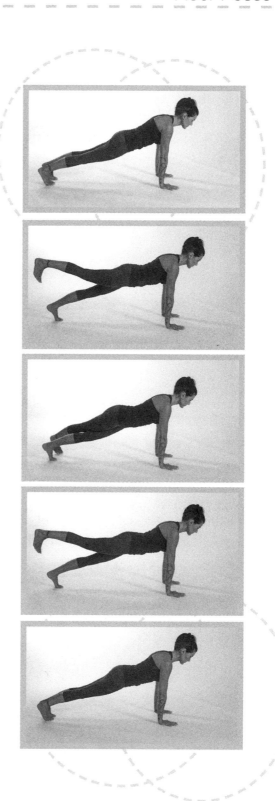

Knee Kissers

In Plank position, draw your right knee in to kiss the right elbow and return to Plank. Switch sides and repeat.

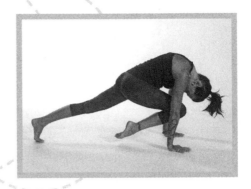

Wrench

In Plank position, keep the stomach firm and externally turn the right wrist up to 180 degrees, or turn it as much as you can until the fingers point straight back. Hold, return, and switch sides. Beginners can drop the knees, turn the wrists, and then pop back up to Plank.

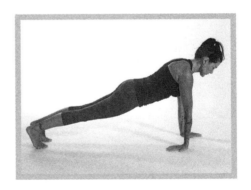

Side Plank

Starting in Plank pose, drop the heels to the right, stacking the feet and engaging the quads. Hold your core tight and extend your left arm to the sky, and hold. If your balance is off you can stagger the feet instead of stacking. Keep lifting through the top hip, push the floor away with the bottom hand, and reach to the sky with the top hand. Repeat on the other side.

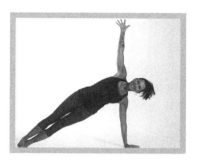

Amens

Starting in Side Plank to the right, hold a weight in your left hand, extend the arm straight up to the sky, lower the arm to the mat, and then return to the extended arm position. Repeat on the other side.

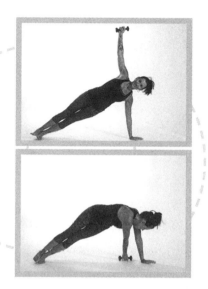

Fan the Fire

From Side Plank, just circle the arm up to the sky, toward the front of your mat, and around your face. Repeat.

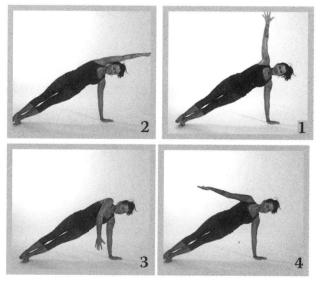

Half Side Plank

Starting in Plank, drop your right knee down and flatten your left foot. Open the body and extend the left arm up to the sky. Your right hand, right lower leg, and left foot should be in one line as though you were on a balance beam. Hold and repeat on the other side. You can also perform Fan the Fire in Half Side Plank for an extra challenge.

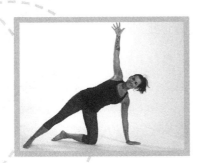

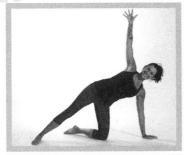

Half Side Plank with Karate Kick

In Half Side Plank, lift the top leg and bend the knee in to meet the elbow of the top arm, then extend the arm and leg and repeat.

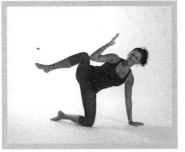

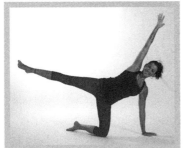

Side Plank with Karate Kick

In Side Plank, lift the top leg and bend the knee in to meet the elbow of the top arm, then extend the arm and leg and repeat.

Cheerleaders

In Side Plank, raise and lower the top leg.

Mountain Climbers

Holding Plank position, press your energy back through your left heel and draw your right knee forward and right foot forward to reach as close as possible to the space between your hands. Return the right leg and do the same on the left, repeat. To increase the difficulty, instead of walking, jump back and forth.

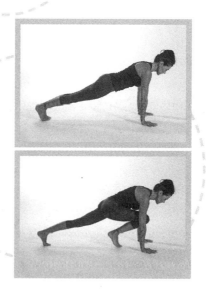

Elbow Me's

In Plank position, grab a weight with your right hand and lift the right hand off the floor with a motion as if you were elbowing someone behind you.

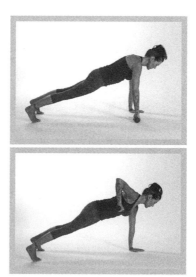

Forearm Plank

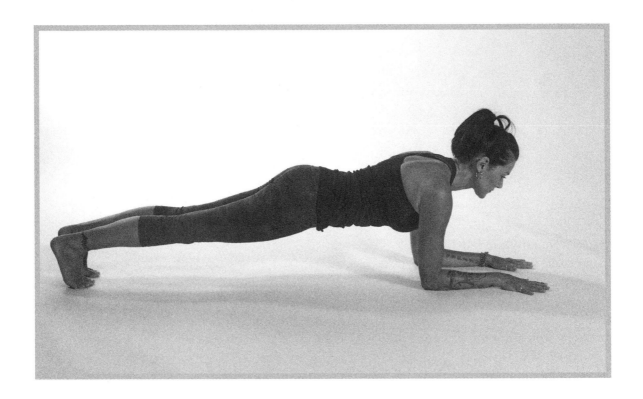

Starting on your hands and knees, lower down to your forearms. Make sure to place your elbows directly under your shoulders and keep your forearms parallel to each other with palms flat. Extend the legs back, tuck the toes, and lift the knees. Your heels should be facing straight up to the sky. Hold. There should not be any pressure or pain in the lower back. To avoid this, tuck the tailbone under and engage the abdominals.

Variations of Forearm Plank

Side Forearm Plank

Starting in Forearm Plank pose, drop your heels to the right then lift your left arm to the sky. Press the floor away with your whole right hand and forearm and lift the hips as high as you can. Hold. Repeat on the other side.

Hip Kisses

Maintaining the Side Forearm Plank pose, keep reaching the left arm to the sky and gently lower your right hip to the floor, kissing the floor and lift it back up. Repeat and do the other side.

Camel

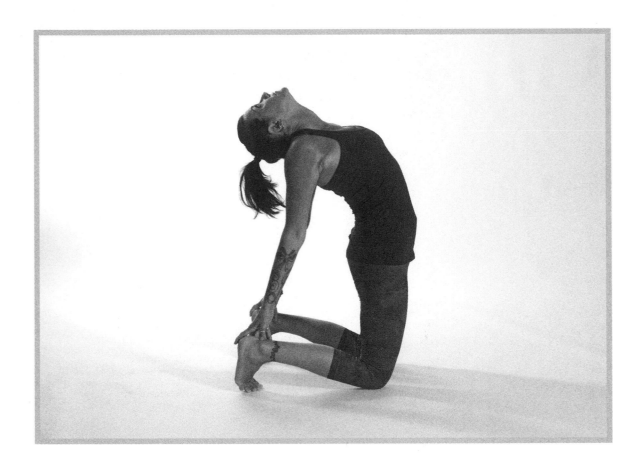

Stand on the knees with the knees hip width apart and toes tucked under, making sure the heels are pointing straight up to the sky. Tuck the tailbone under to relieve any back pressure. Lift the arms up to the sky and with a windmill rotation of the right arm, bring the right hand to the right heel. Press the hips forward and do the same with the left hand. Feel that you are pressing the hips forward, lifting the heart up and, if possible, dropping the head back.

Camel Praise

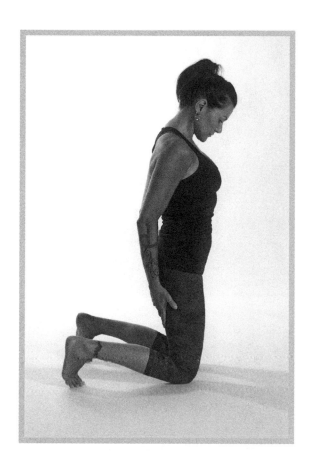 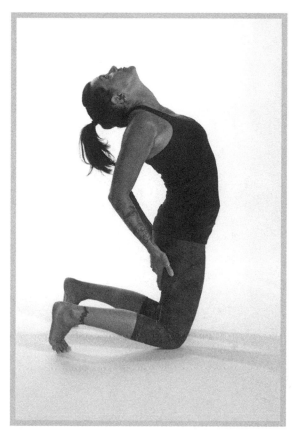

Starting in Camel position, have your arms down by your side and from the waist up, lift up and perform a back bend. From the waist down, press the hips forward. Return to starting position and repeat as many times as needed.

Quad Crunch

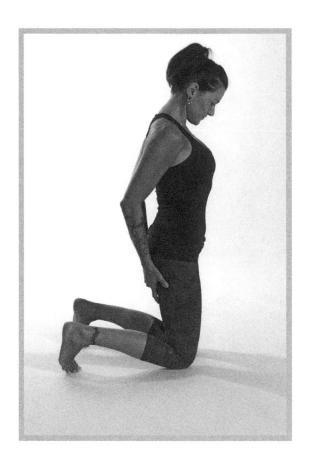 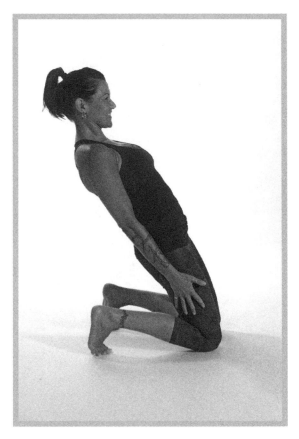

Starting in Camel position, have your arms down by your side and lean back, hinging the body from the knee joint. Once you cannot go any farther, break at the waist and press down through the lower leg and press back up to starting position.

Upward Dog

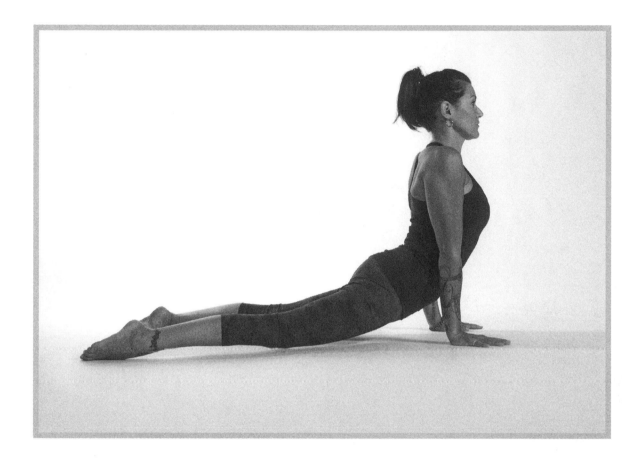

Lie down on your belly with palms facing down and fingers spread flat, directly under your shoulder joints. Start to press the arms straight and raise the body off the floor. At the same time push the tops of the feet into the floor. The only parts of your body touching the floor in Upward Dog are the tops of the feet and the hands. Press your chest forward and pull your shoulders back. Tuck the tailbone, engage the legs, and hold. If you experience back pain, it is likely that your hands are too far forward and you need to make sure once you are extended in the pose that the wrists are directly under your shoulders.

Table

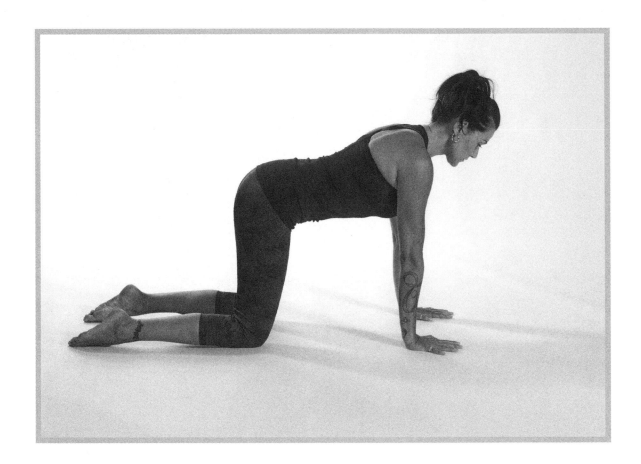

Table is simply assuming the position of being on your hands and knees. The important thing to remember is to keep your wrist joints directly under your shoulders and your knees directly under your hips.

Variations of Table

3-Legged Table

Starting in Table, extend one leg back straight out from its own hip. Repeat on the other side.

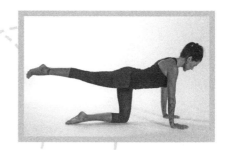

Folding Table Cross-Over

From 3-Legged Table, with the right leg extended back, bend the right knee, and drop the right knee over and behind the left leg. Have the right knee touch the ground and then return it back. Repeat on the other side.

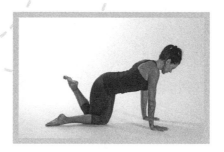

Table Scissors

From 3-Legged Table, with the right leg extended back, keep the leg straight and bring the right leg behind and over the left leg until the right toes touch the floor, then return it back. Repeat on the other side.

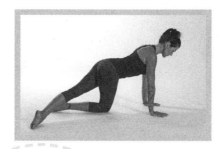

Clock Holds

Starting in Table, lift the right leg straight up behind you until it is hip height. Flex the right foot and externally rotate the whole leg until the right foot is now at a 3 o'clock position. Return it back. When doing this on the left leg, the left foot will be at a 9 o'clock position.

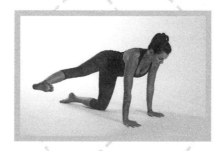

Inverted Table

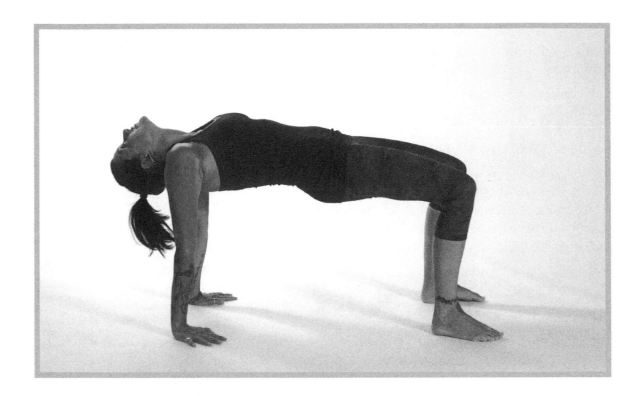

Starting in a seated position, bring your hands behind you on the floor, shoulder-width apart with palms flat and fingers spread. Turn the fingers to face you. Bend the knees and on an inhale, lift the hips off the floor to hip height by pressing equally into the hands and feet, then drop the hips back down to the floor.

Child's Pose

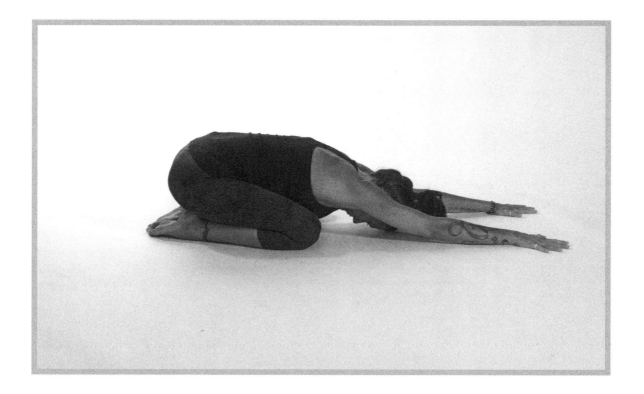

On your hands and knees, pull the hips all the way back until your hips touch your heels, or as close as you can reach. Extend the arms forward along the floor with palms facing down, and rest your head on the floor.

Squats

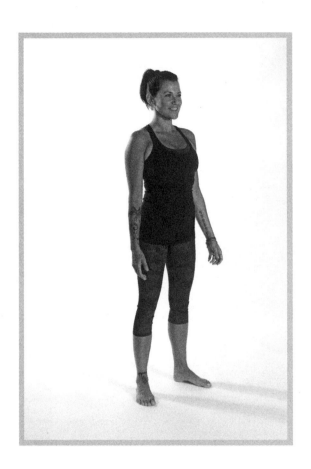
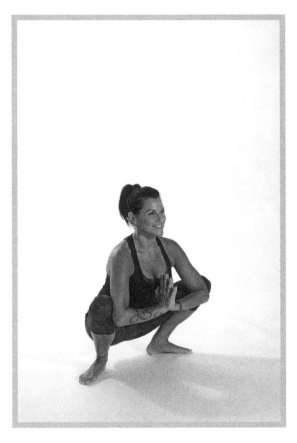

Set your feet hips-width apart and allow your feet to point in the direction they are most comfortable in (what is most important is that the knees point in the same direction as the feet). Bend the knees and sink down as far as you can go, as long as your feet are flat. Hold. Try to keep a flat back and bend your elbows and press them against the inner knee while your hands are in prayer pose.

Variations of Squat

Rockets

Maintaining all the precision Squats, move from Squat to standing and keep repeating.

Take-Offs

Using the same positioning as Squats, instead of raising up to standing, use more power and jump up and get off the floor briefly, then return to Squat. Repeat.

Plié Squat

Take your feet a little wider than hips-width apart and turn the toes out approximately 45 degrees. Bend the knees, keeping them pointing directly over the toes until the knees are at a 90-degree angle, then return to standing.

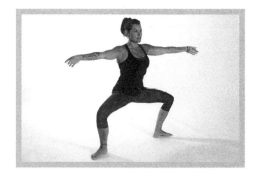

Toe Balance Squat

Keep the legs together and bend the knees, sinking down until you are sitting on the heels. With this variation of squat, your feet are not flat; the heels will rise up. Squeeze the inner thighs together, hold.

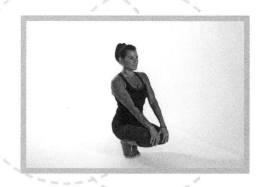

Cobra

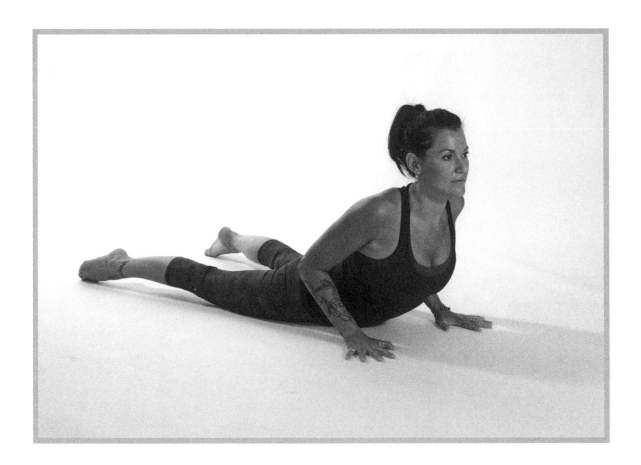

Lie face down on the floor. Stretch your legs back, with the tops of the feet on the floor. Place your hands on the floor under your shoulders, with fingers spread and palms flat. Draw the elbows back in toward your body. On an inhalation, begin to straighten the arms to lift the chest off the floor, going only to the height at which you can maintain a connection through your hips all the way down to your toes. Press the tailbone toward the floor. Firm the shoulder blades against the back and pull the heart forward. Lift through the top of the chest. Hold.

Variations of Cobra

Cobra Push-Up

Lift into Cobra, and then lower back down to the chest. Be sure that you keep the elbows tight to the body, pointing behind you at all times. Inhale as you come up and exhale as you lower down.

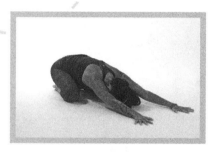

Slither

Starting in Cobra, lower down to the chest. Keep the hands and feet exactly where they are, do not move them. As though you are rolling a ball with your chin back toward your knees, lift the hips high and keep the head low, pushing firmly into the hands and using your arm strength until you are all the way back to Child's Pose. Then as though you are rolling a ball forward with your nose, keep the head low and hips high and return back to Cobra. Repeat.

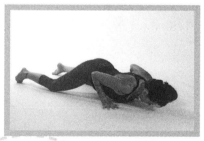

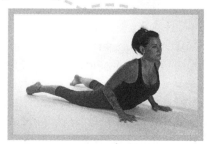

Inverted Plank

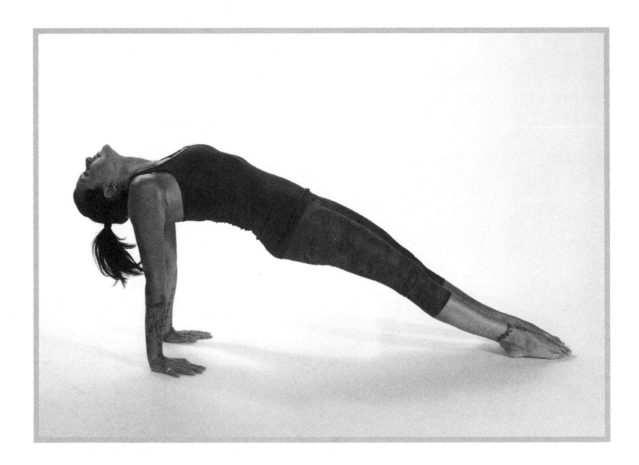

Sitting on the floor with your legs extended out straight in front of you, rest back on your hands with your fingers pointing toward your body. Keep the palms flat with fingers spread and hands shoulder-width apart. Press down through your hands and through your heels to lift the entire body off the floor until your arms are straight. Keep the legs straight and internally rotate the thighs, pointing the feet until someday your big toes touch the floor. To protect your wrists, it is important that you plug the whole hand firmly into the floor.

Variations of Inverted Plank

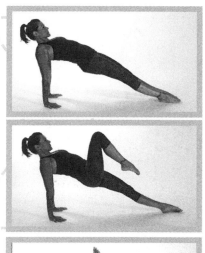

Rockettes

Starting in Inverted Plank, lift the right leg off the floor, bend the right knee into your chest, extend the right leg straight up to the sky, and then lower to the starting position. Repeat on the other side.

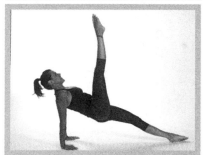

Shark Attack

While you are in Inverted Plank, maintain hip height, place sliders under your heels, and slide the heels apart as far as you can and back together.

For beginners, lifting the hip high may be too challenging. In this case, lift the hips as high as you can until you build up more and more strength.

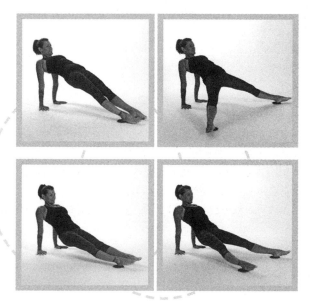

Face Down Snow Angel

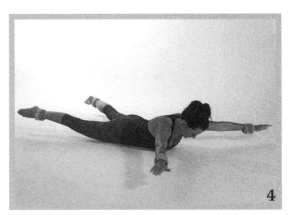

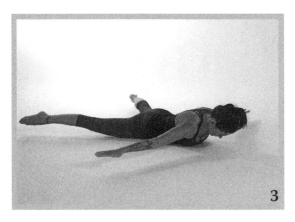

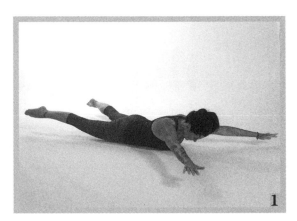

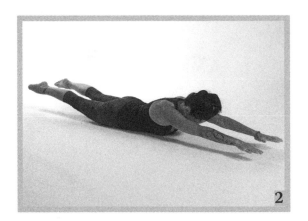

Lying down on your stomach, use your back muscles and lift the legs and arms off the floor about an inch, mimicking the movement you would do if you were making a snow angel (essentially a face-down, lying down jumping jack movement). To avoid overextending the head or stressing the neck, lift only enough so that your face is still looking down but not touching the floor.

Locust

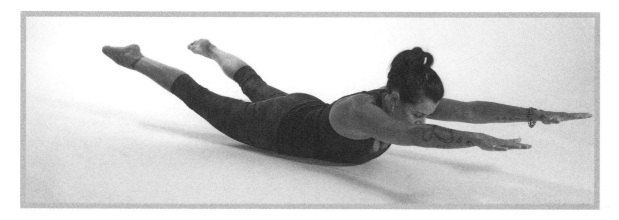

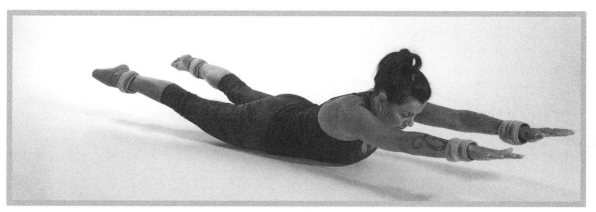

Lying face down on your stomach, reach your arms over your head and lift the arms and legs off the floor as high as you can, making a "C" shape with your body. For an extra challenge, you can perform this movement using wrist weights and ankle weights.

Canoes

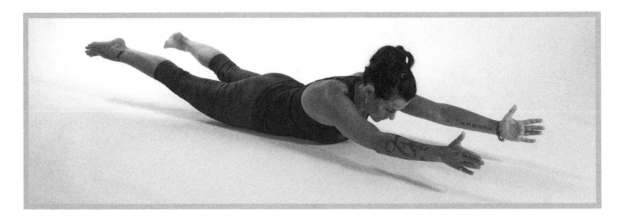

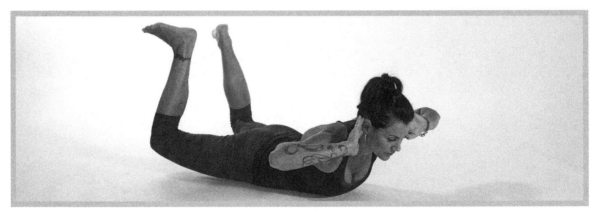

Starting in Locust pose, bend the knees at a 90-degree angle and flex your feet. Pulse the legs up to the sky. Bend the elbow and place your hands behind your head.

Bow

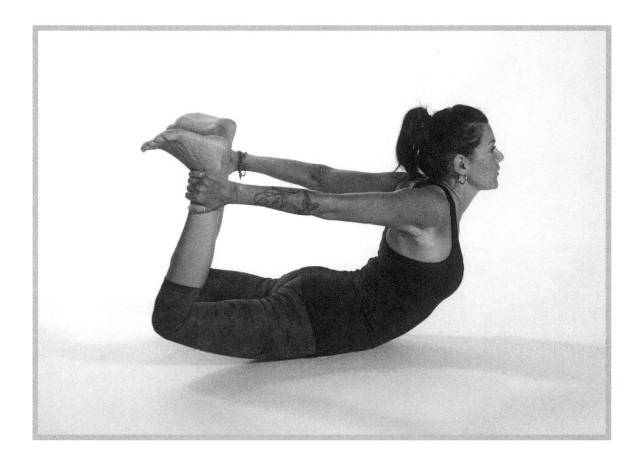

Lie down on your stomach, bend your knees, and reach around to grab the ankles on each leg. Flex your feet, relax your back, and press your feet back as much as you can. This movement will lift the upper body up high, with the chest facing the front of your mat. Once you are in this position, keep pressing the legs back and at the same time lift your feet up to try to get the thighs off the floor as well. Hold and breathe. Slowly lower down onto your stomach.

Bridge

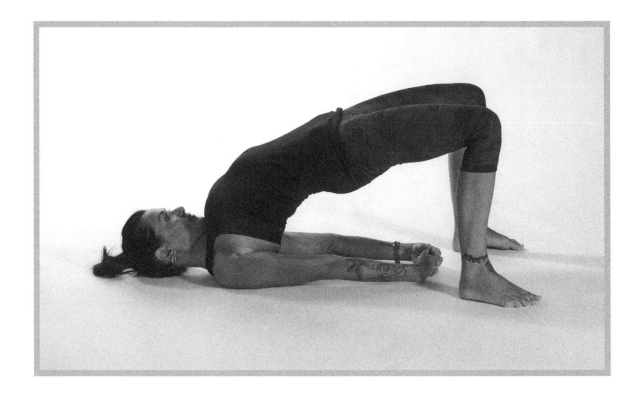

Lying down on your back with your knees bent and feet flat on the floor, push down into your feet and lift your hips up off the floor as high as you can. Snuggle the shoulders under you toward each other and interlace your fingers if you are able. Hold.

Variations of Bridge

Bridge Lifts

Get into Bridge position with hips lifted, pause, and then lower the hips back down, and keep repeating.

Daddy Long Legs

In Bridge, hold the hips high then draw the right knee into your chest, straighten it up to the sky, then lower it down to an inch away from the floor, bend the knee in, and repeat on the other side.

Dragonfly

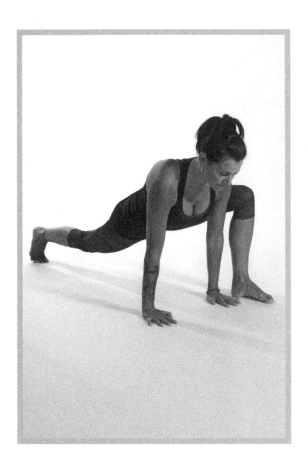 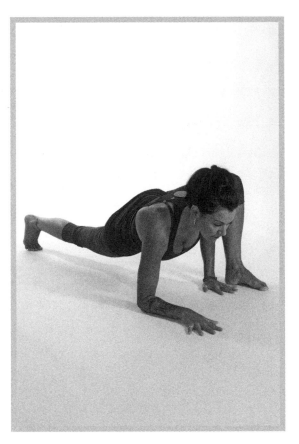

Place your legs in a lunge position, with the right leg forward and right knee bent 90 degrees, with the right foot flat on the floor. Extend your left leg back straight with toes tucked under and your left heel facing straight up to the sky. Place your hands on the floor on the inside of the right leg with palms flat and fingers spread. If you are able, rest on your left forearm while maintaining the lunge positioning, and lower to both forearms. Hold. Repeat on the other side.

Seals

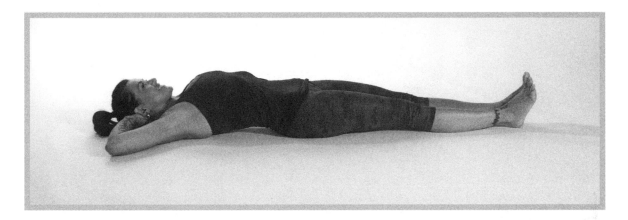

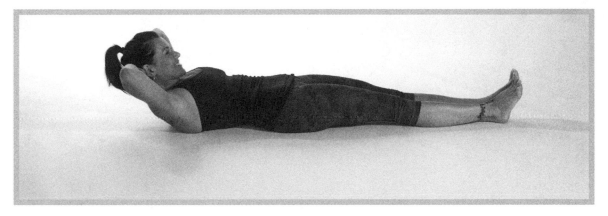

Lying down on your back with your legs extended and straight out in front of you, gently squeeze your inner thighs together. Place your hands behind your head, ground your lower body, and lift your upper body up off the floor. Try to have your mid-back lifted off the floor. Pause, lower, and repeat.

Twisted Root Abdominals

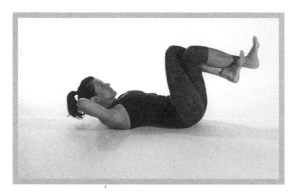
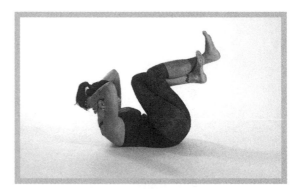
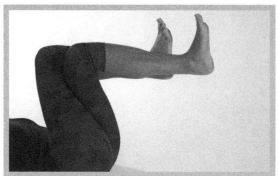
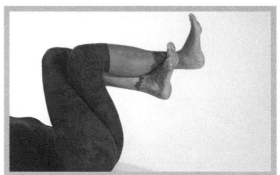

Lie on your back and bend your knees, with the feet flat on the floor. Cross the right thigh over the left thigh, gently squeezing the inner thighs together. If you are able, continue to wrap your right lower leg under the left to wrap the right foot under the left ankle. Lift your feet off the floor, place your hands behind your head, and as you bring the upper body off the floor at the same time lift the knees toward your face and lift the hips off the floor for a quick squeeze. Release and repeat on the other side.

For those who have a difficult time hooking the foot or if you have problematic knees, just cross the thighs and squeeze the inner thighs together.

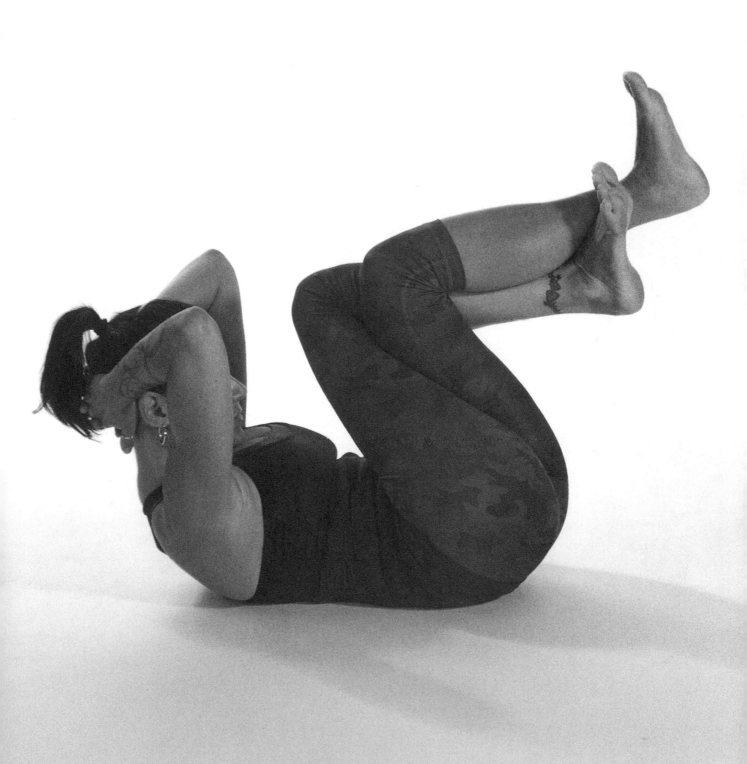

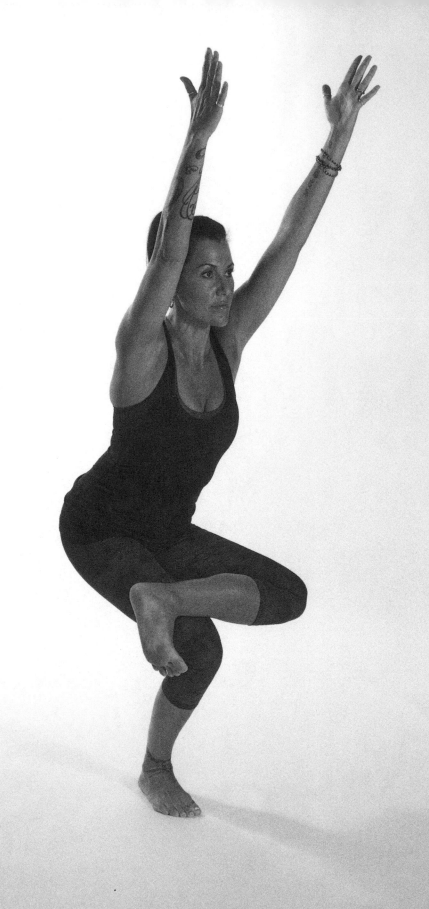

Standing Poses

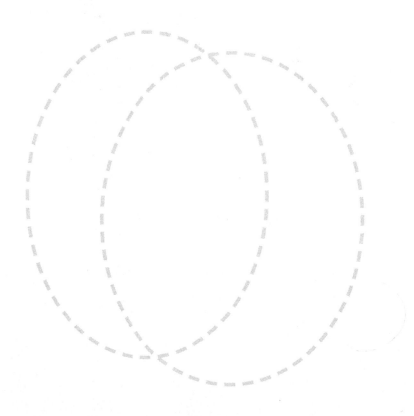

Band Side Step

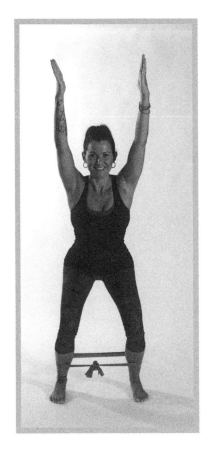 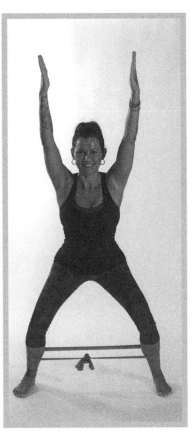 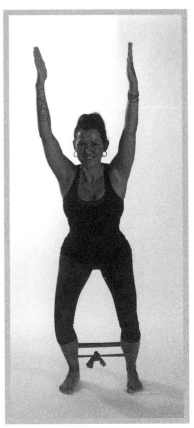

Stand with a band around the lower legs, creating enough tension so that the band does not slide down. Bend the knees and keep the back flat and extended. Maintain the tension in the band and step to the side and back.

High Knees

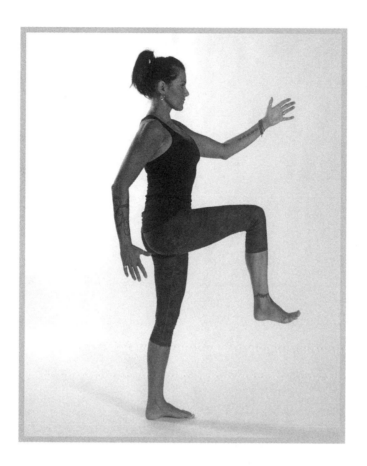

Stand in an exaggerated walking movement, raising your right knee high, returning the foot back down, and then raising your left knee high. Repeat.

Butt Kicks

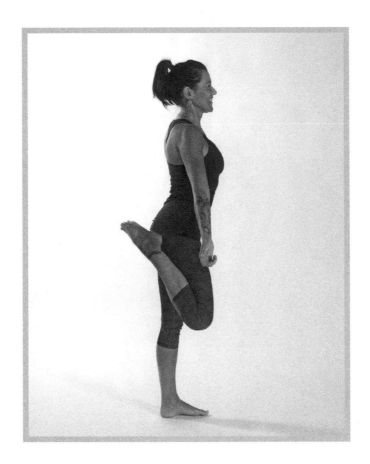

Standing, bend the right knee with enough force to gently kick the right butt cheek, switch sides, and repeat on the other side.

Serpentine Jump

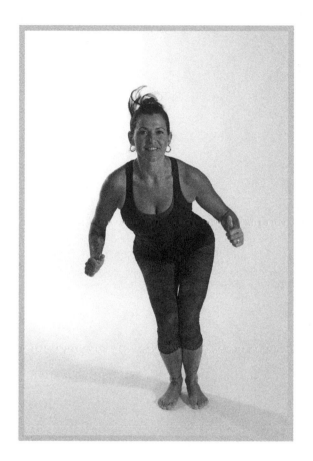 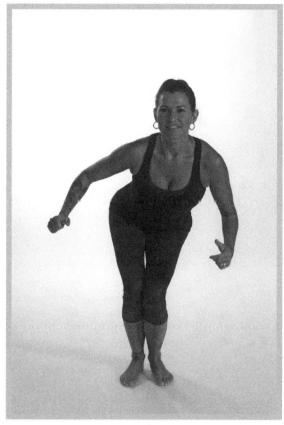

Stand with your feet together and knees slightly bent. Keep your arms down by your side with the elbows slightly bent. (This will resemble a skier's stance.) Bend the knees and while keeping the knees and inner thighs connected, jump with a two-foot take-off to the right, jump back to center, jump left, and then back to center again. Repeat.

Wall Squat

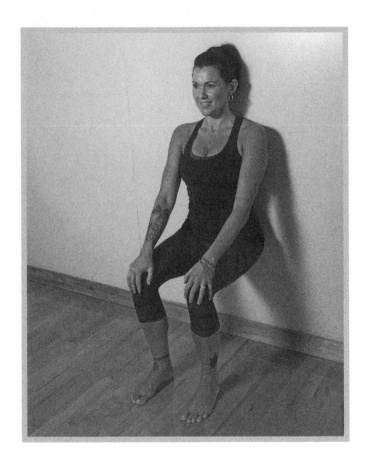

Standing against a wall with your feet about hips-width apart and parallel, walk the feet about 2 feet away from the wall. Slide the back down the wall until your thighs are parallel to the floor and your knees are in a 90-degree angle, and hold.

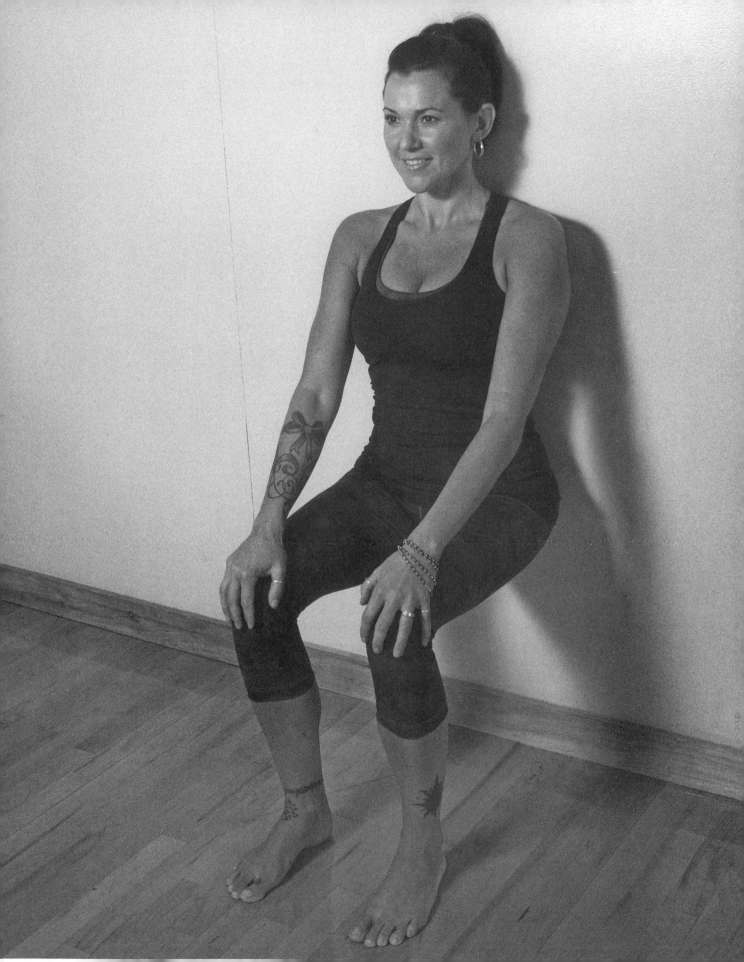

Runner's Lunge

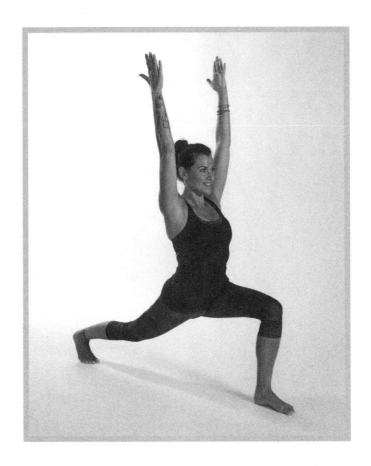

Move your right foot forward until your knee can hit a 90-degree angle and your foot is flat, with your back leg long and straight. Your left toes should be tucked under and your heel pointing straight up to the sky. At the same time, extend your arms straight up to the sky with no bend in the elbow. Place your palms facing each other with the upper arms alongside the sides of your head as much as possible. Hold, distributing your weight evenly between the front foot and the back leg, foot, and heel. Repeat on the other side.

Variations of Runner's Lunge

Knee Floor Kissers

Starting in Runner's Lunge with your right leg forward in a 90-degree angle, dip the left knee to the floor to "kiss" the floor and repeat. Repeat on the other side.

On Your Marks

Holding the Runner's Lunge position, push off the back toes and foot, lurching your whole body forward and then back. Keep the right knee in a 90-degree angle the whole time; you are not coming up and down; the energy of the pose is forward and back. Repeat on the other side.

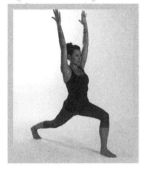 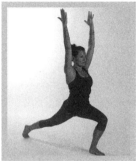

SOS

Holding the Runner's Lunge position, bring your arms up and down at your sides to imitate a jumping jack movement. Repeat on the other side.

Pinwheels

Holding the Runner's Lunge position, bring your arms down to a 90-degree angle at your sides, and keep your lower body still. While holding a strong lunge position, twist the upper body like a pinwheel. Repeat on the other side.

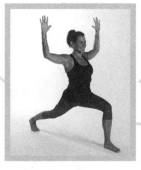 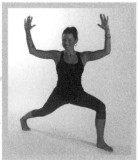

Stop Traffic

Holding the Runner's Lunge position, extend your arms straight out to the sides from your shoulders. Flex the wrists hard so your fingers are pointing straight up and your palms are facing out to "stop traffic."

Lunge Twist

In Runner's Lunge, bring your hands into prayer position at the center of your chest (also known as the heart center). With the right leg forward, bring the left elbow to the outside of the right thigh. Push the arm against the thigh and press the prayer into the heart center as you extend the heart through. Hold, constantly dropping the shoulders away from the ears and twisting deeper and deeper. Keep a lot of weight back through the left heel and keep the back leg straight. Turn your chin over the right shoulder the best you can. Repeat on the other side.

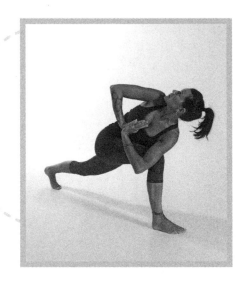

Crescent Lunge

Assume the same position as the Runner's Lunge, but drop the back knee down to the floor and untuck the back toes. Repeat on the other side.

Crescent Lunge Twist

From Crescent Lunge position, bring your hands to the heart center in prayer, similar to the Lunge Twist. Bring your left elbow to the outside of the right thigh and twist. Use the left elbow against the right thigh for torque to twist deeper and deeper. Gently turn your chin over your right shoulder, keep the shoulders away from the ears, and once you feel steady, press the hips forward. Hold. Repeat on the other side.

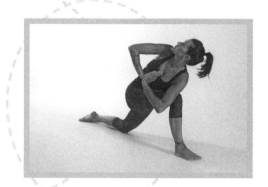

Crescent Lunge Hammie Curl

Come into the Crescent Lunge position, with your right leg forward and left knee down with the left toes untucked. Keep extending the upper body up and the hips forward, then start to bend the left leg as much and you can and return it to the floor. Repeat on the other side. In the beginning this can be tough on the knee, so you may want to add some extra cushioning under the knee.

Half Side Squat

From Crescent Lunge position with your right leg forward, put your hands on the floor on the inside of the right leg and start to twist your body until you are facing to the left. As you turn, rotate your left leg so the left toes point straight up to the sky (your right leg will be in a half squat). Bend the right knee as much as you can, while keeping the right foot flat. Make sure your right knee tracks in the same direction as your right toes. Repeat on the other side.

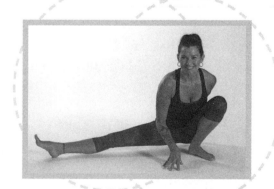

Standing Straddle Forward Bend

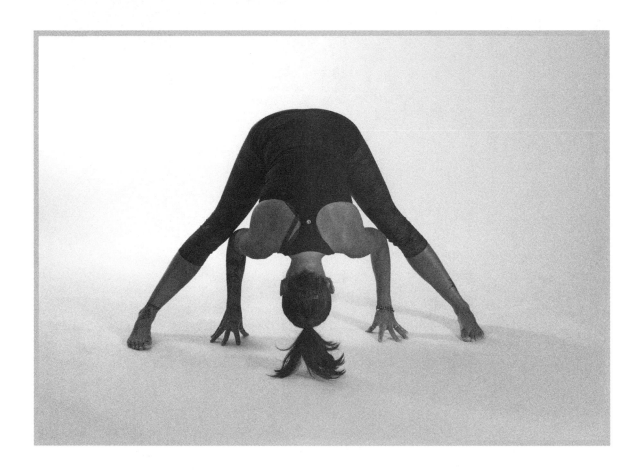

Stand in a wide leg stance so that the distance between your feet is approximately the length of one of your legs. Make sure your feet are parallel to each other and you are pressing down through your whole foot equally, instead of rolling out on the outer edge of your foot. Extend the arms out from your shoulders parallel to the floor and hold. Fold yourself over from your hips, not from your spine.

If you would like to take it to the next level, grab the opposite elbow with the opposite hand and drape a sandbag over your forearms. This will significantly help you to stretch the hamstrings and open the shoulders.

Variation of Standing Straddle Forward Bend

Genies

Stand in the prep pose for Standing Straddle Forward Bend with your arms extended out from the shoulders. Bend the elbows and place the right hand on top of the back of the left hand. Hold your hands at chest height. From here, hinge over from the hips to fold over with the back flat. With the back rounded, roll back up one vertebra at a time. Repeat.

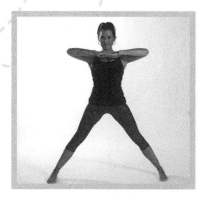

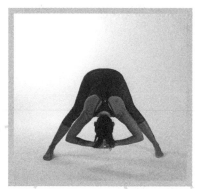

Triangle

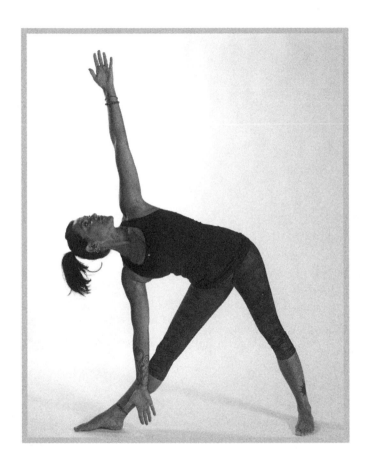

Stand with both legs straight, in a wide leg stance so that the distance between your feet is approximately the length of one of your legs. Turn the right toes out 90 degrees and turn the left foot in slightly. Extend your arms up to shoulder height, reach your energy through your right hand, and start to slide the back of the right hand down the inside of the right leg. Stop when you feel resistance, breathe, and repeat on the other side when appropriate.

Variations of Triangle Pose

Triangle Flags

While holding Triangle pose (to the right), reach the left arm up to the sky and bring it over your left ear until your left upper arm is right next to the left ear. Hold. Rotate the left palm to face the floor. Hold. Take it one step further by bringing the right arm up parallel to the floor until the right palm and the left palm come together in prayer. Repeat on the other side.

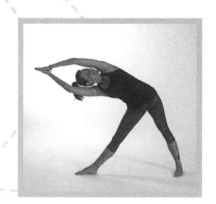

Revolving Triangle

Hold the same foot position as Triangle pose. Turn the hips to face the direction of the right toes so that your hips, torso, and shoulders are facing forward. Soften the right knee and fold over from the hips into a flat back. The left hand will be on the inside of the right foot, on the right foot, or on the outside of the right foot. Place it strong and secure. With the right hand on your right hip and keeping the hips square to the front, start to twist to the right and open the chest to the right. If you can, release the right hand up to the sky, palm facing the wall like the chest. Push down through the left hand, extend the torso, and twist. If possible, straighten the right leg and hold. Repeat on the other side.

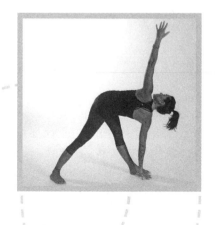

Standing Mountain

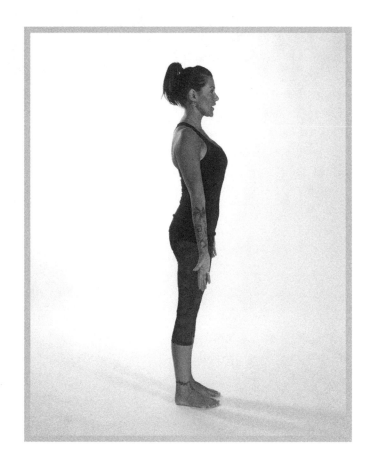

Stand with both feet together, keeping the body tall and extended. Keep the arms down by your side with palms facing forward, in a simple neutral standing position.

Variations of Mountain Pose

Standing Backbend

With your legs in Standing Mountain pose, extend the arms out and up over your head, keeping the arms shoulders-width apart and palms facing each other. Lengthen your side body, engage your legs, firm up the glutes, and lift the heart and chest up, then start to backbend until you feel resistance. Hold and breathe.

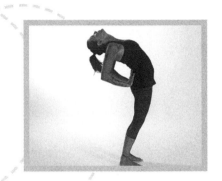

Hold the Bundle

In Standing Mountain pose, bend the right knee into your chest and hold. Switch when suggested. For an extra challenge, you can perform this movement using ankle weights.

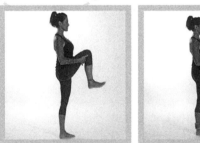

Deliver the Bundle

From the position of Holding the Bundle, grab the right bent leg behind the thigh with both hands, extend the right leg straight out in front of you, and use the hands to hold the leg or release the hands for more of a challenge. For added difficulty, you can perform this movement using ankle weights.

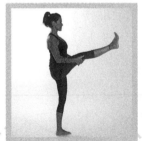
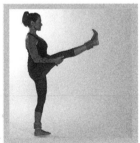

Step-Ups

Step your right foot up onto a stable bench at approximately knee height, then follow with the left foot. Step the right foot down and the left foot follows. On the next round, step with the left foot first.

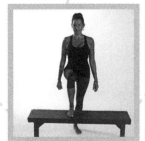
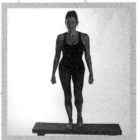

Cross-Kicks

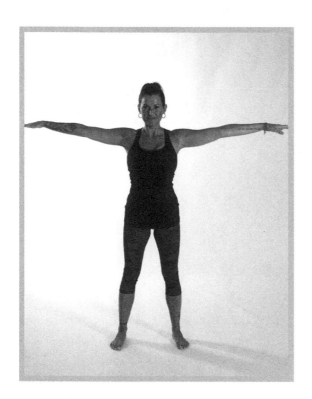 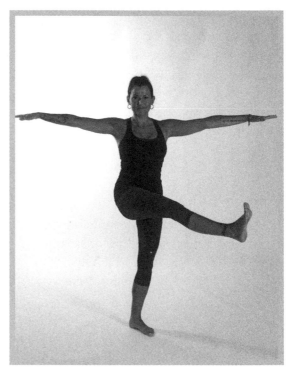

Standing with your feet shoulder-width apart, extend your arms out from your shoulders, keeping your arms parallel to the floor. Start to kick the legs across the body, alternating legs.

Variation of Cross-Kicks

Karate Kicks

In the same stance as the Cross-Kicks, bend the left knee and keep all of your weight in the left leg as you side kick with the right leg.

Spar

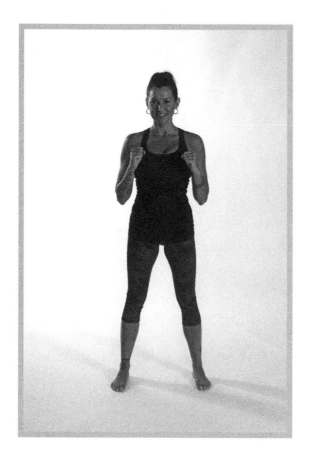 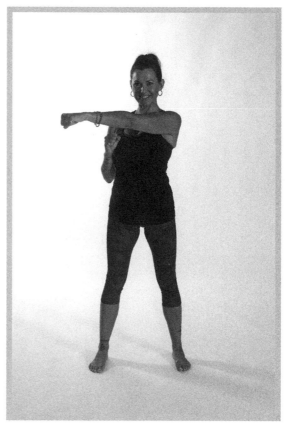

Stand with your legs shoulder-width apart with the arms up, elbows bent, and fists resting gently on the chest. On each exhale, punch across the body and return to starting position, then alternate.

Warrior 1

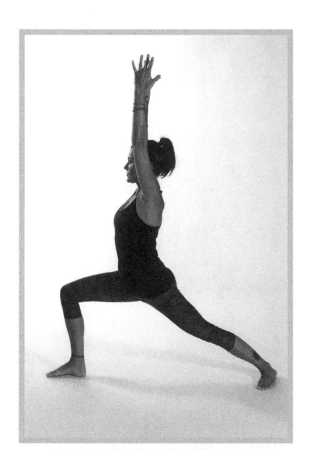 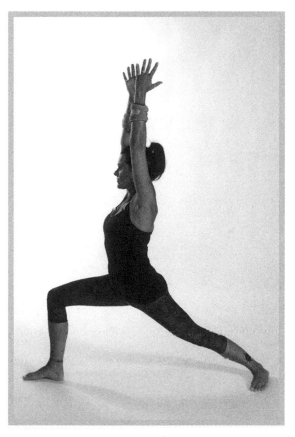

Step your right foot forward, and bend the right knee to a 90-degree angle. Extend the left leg back fully with a straight knee. Flatten the left foot until the left toes point out at approximately a 45-degree angle. Direct the front knee to point straight ahead over the right toes and reach your arms straight up to the sky with palms facing each other. Be sure while holding the pose that the hips are pointing straight ahead. If your hips are tight, position your feet to make this possible. Full expression of this pose is when your right heel and left foot are aligned; however, it is more important to have the hips and torso squared to the front of the mat than to position the feet in the full expression of the pose. Hold and breathe. Repeat on the other side. For an extra challenge, you can perform this movement using wrist weights.

Warrior 2

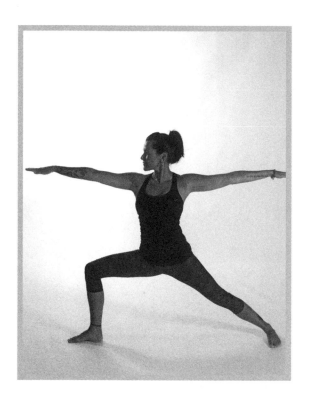
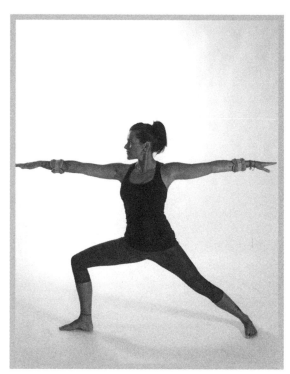

Stand with the feet approximately 3 feet apart and turn the right foot forward 90-degrees and the left foot in about 45-degrees. Bend the right knee until it creates a 90-degree angle and extend the arms out from the shoulders until they are parallel to the floor, with palms facing the floor. Look over the right shoulder, hold. Repeat on the other side. For an extra challenge, you can perform this movement using wrist weights.

Variation of Warrior 2

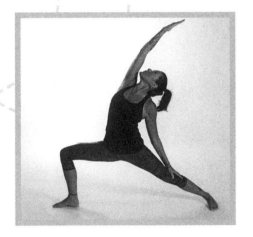

Reverse Warrior

In Warrior 2 position, turn the right palm up to the sky and slide the left hand down the back of the left leg. Raise the right arm up and over your head as far as you can, while sliding the left hand down as far as you can, then hold. Repeat on the other side. For an extra challenge, you can perform this movement using wrist weights.

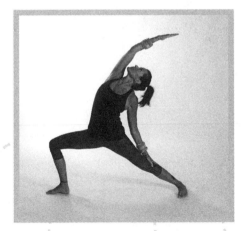

Warrior 3

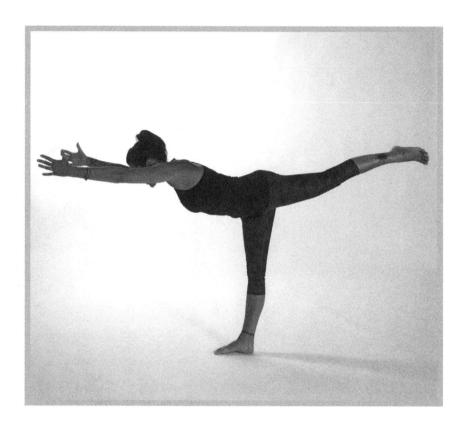

Starting in Standing Mountain pose, extend the arms over your head with palms facing each other. Hinge your body from the hips, lowering the upper body and raising one leg like a see-saw until your body is as close to parallel as possible. Hold. Repeat on the other side. For an extra challenge, you can perform this movement using wrist weights, as shown on the next page.

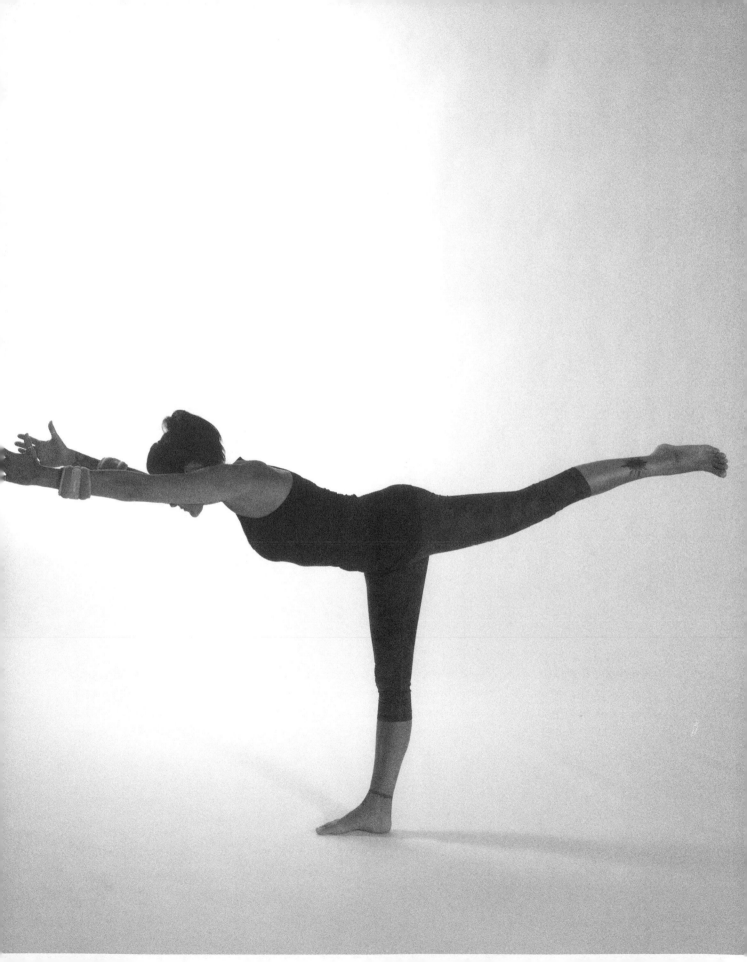

Standing Forward Bend

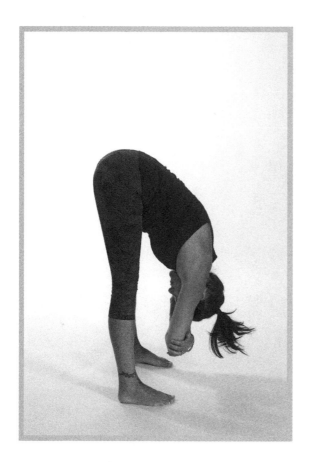 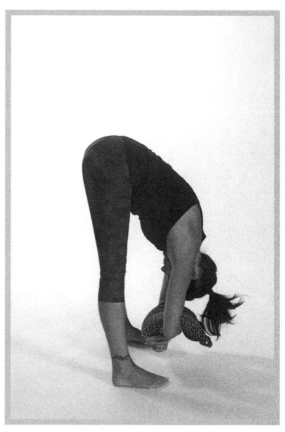

Set your feet hips-width apart with the feet grounded. Fold over from the hips and grab the opposite arm with the opposite elbow. Hold. If this stretch is felt more in the back than in the hamstrings, then soften the knees. For an extra challenge, you can perform this movement using a sandbag.

Variations of Standing Forward Bend

Standing Split

In the same position as the Standing Forward Bend, place the fingertips to the floor in front of the feet and raise one leg as high as you can up to the sky. Hold and repeat on the other side.

Split Kicks

From Standing Forward Bend, place the fingertips on the floor in front of the feet and kick the right leg up to the sky like a Standing Split, quickly return the leg, and switch to the other side. Continue for suggested amount of time.

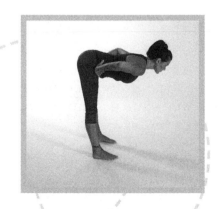

Halfway-Up Flat Back

From Standing Forward Bend, put your hands on your hips and bring the back halfway up until it is parallel to the floor. Lengthen the spine, hold, and breathe.

Jumping Jacks

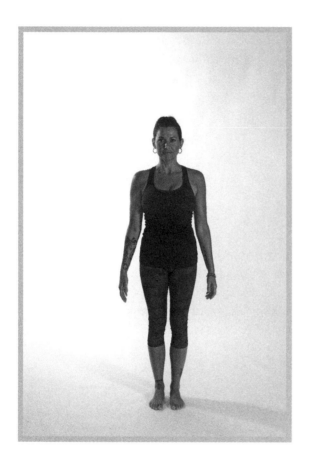 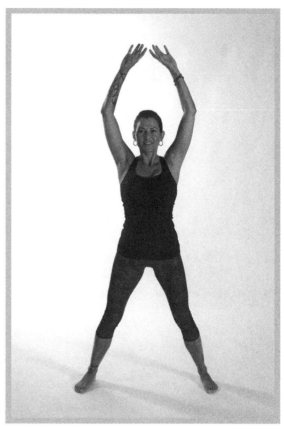

Starting in a standing position with your arms down by your sides, jump your feet shoulder-width apart and at the same time swing your arms up over your head. Jump the feet back together and return the arms down to your sides. Repeat.

Faux Jump Rope

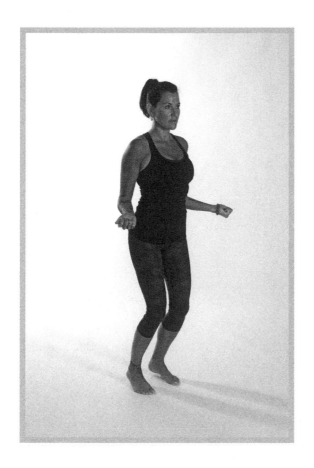 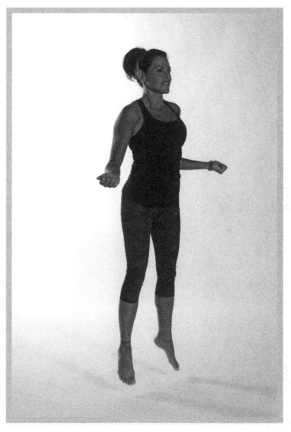

Perform the same movement as you would with a jump rope, but without using a jump rope. Move the arms at your side as if you were holding a jump rope. This provides the same great exercise, but with no stress about missing the jumps.

Yoga Burpees

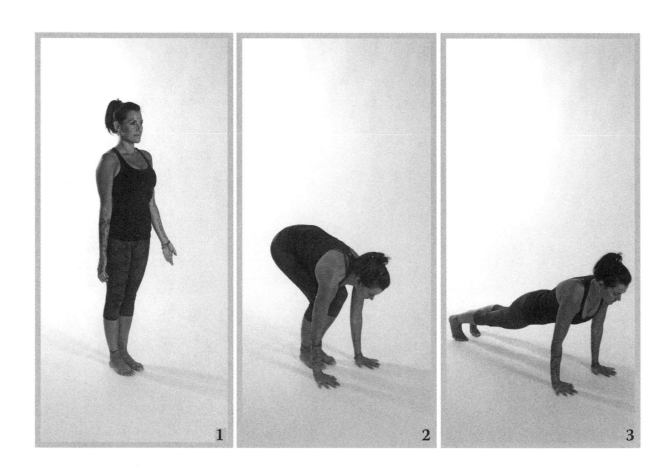

Start in Standing Mountain pose at the front of your mat. Fold to Standing Forward Bend. Plant the hands on the floor and jump back to Plank pose (or the top position of a push-up). Lower into a push-up. Return to Plank pose. Jump the feet back to Standing Forward Bend and return to Standing Mountain pose. Repeat.

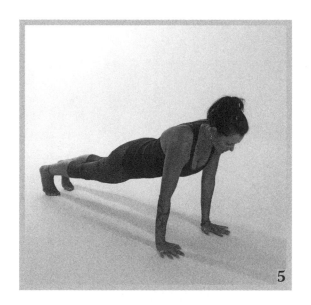

5

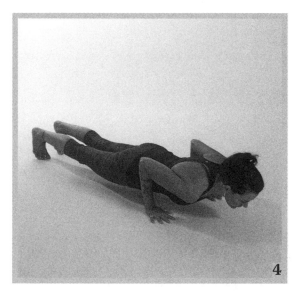

4

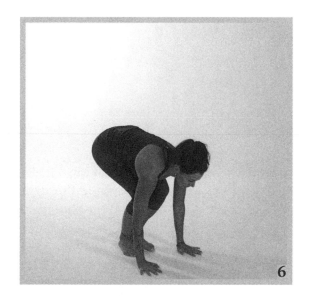

6

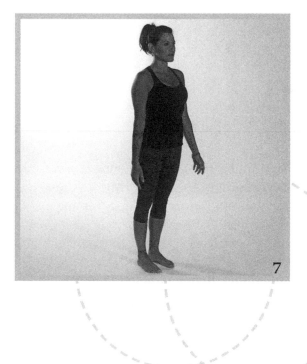

7

Right Angle

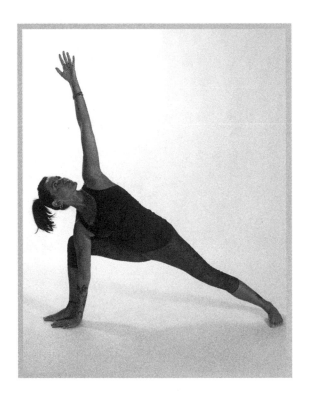 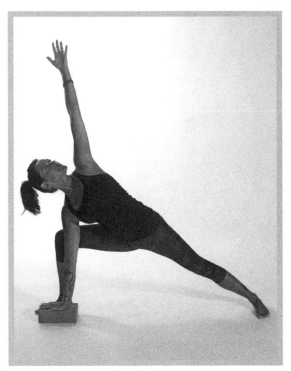

Standing sideways on the mat with your feet 3 to 4 feet apart, turn the right foot forward 90 degrees, pointing to the front of the mat. Turn the back foot in 45 degrees. Bend the right knee until it creates a 90-degree angle and extend the arms straight out from the shoulders with palms facing the ground. Tilt over until you can place your hand on the floor or a block on the inside of the right foot. Bring the left arm straight up to the sky. Hold. Repeat on the other side.

Variations of Right Angle

Right Angle Fan the Fire

Holding the Right Angle pose, instead of straightening the left arm up to the sky, start to rotate the arm clockwise, in front of your face, down toward the ground, and back up again, repeating. Repeat on the other side.

Right Angle Flag

While holding Right Angle pose (to the right), reach the left arm up to the sky and bring it over your left ear until your left upper arm is right next to the left ear. Hold. Rotate the left palm to face the floor. Hold. Take it one step further by bringing the right arm up parallel to the floor until the right palm and the left palm come together in a prayer position. Repeat on the other side.

Chair

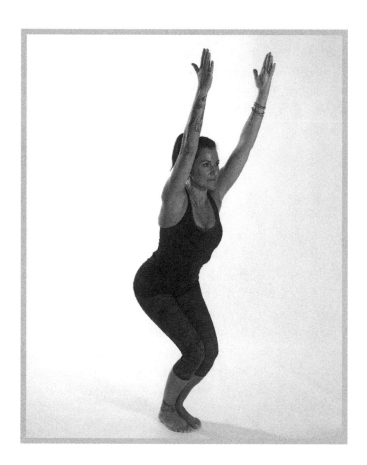

Start in Standing Mountain pose and lift the arms up to the sky with palms facing each other. Keeping the back flat, bend the knees and "sit" into the pose as far as you can with the feet remaining flat on the floor. Keep the chest facing the front of the room with the chin in a neutral position. Squeeze the inner thighs together and hold.

Variations of Chair

Side to Side Chair

Hold Chair pose and step side to side. For increased difficulty, place a workout band around the ankles and keep the tension.

Chair Twists

Starting in Chair pose, bring the hands into the center of the chest and place the left elbow on the outside of the right knee, pushing the left arm against the thigh to create more torque to twist. Keep the knees together and facing forward while maintaining the bend in the knees. Hold. Repeat on the other side.

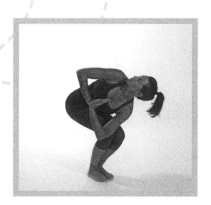

Figure 4 Chair

While in Chair pose, bring the left lower leg across the right thigh, flex the left foot, and hold. Repeat on the other side.

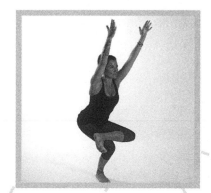

Figure 4 Chair Fold

While in Figure 4 Chair pose, bring the left lower leg across the right thigh, flex the left foot, and hold. Fold over and touch the floor. Repeat on the other side.

Eagle

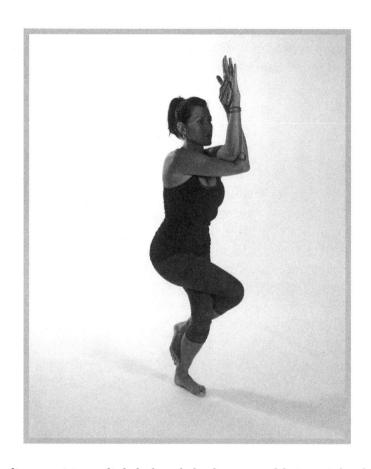

Starting in a standing position, slightly bend the knees and bring right thigh over the left thigh as though you were crossing your legs in a chair. If you can, wrap the right lower leg around and tuck the right foot behind the left calf. If that is not possible, just squeeze the inner thighs together. Extend the arms out from your shoulders and bring the arms together in front of you with the right arm under the left arm, bending the elbows 90 degrees so that the thumbs are positioned as they would poke you in the face. Continue wrapping the arms around through the forearms until your palms are pressed together. Drop your shoulders away from your ears, lift the elbows up to shoulder height, and press the hands away from the face until you feel a shoulder stretch. Hold, then repeat on the opposite side.

Variations of Eagle

Eagle Lunge

Start in a lunge position with the right leg forward and left leg extended back. Position your arms into Eagle pose, with the right arm under the left arm. Hold. Repeat on the other side.

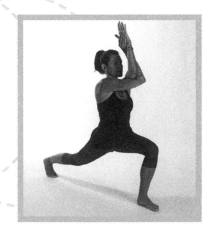

Skaters

Stand on the right foot with the right knee slightly bent. Slide the left toes behind you and to the right to a 5 o'clock position, bending your right knee enough while you do this so that you can touch the floor with your left hand. Slide the left foot back and repeat on the opposite side.

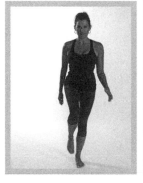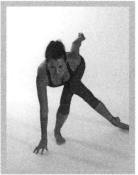

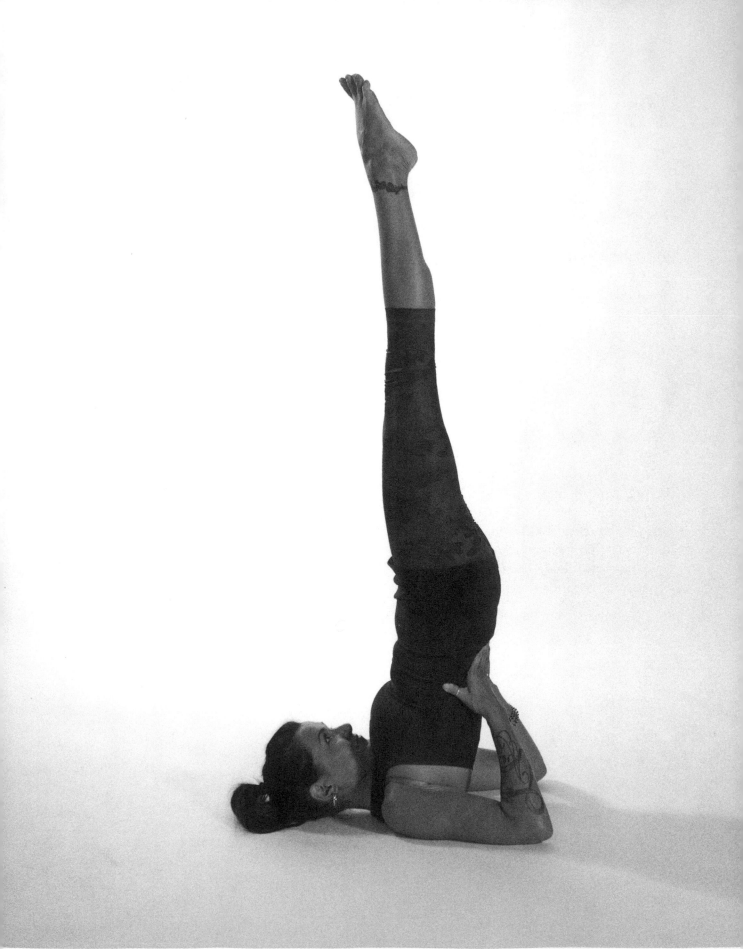

Inversions

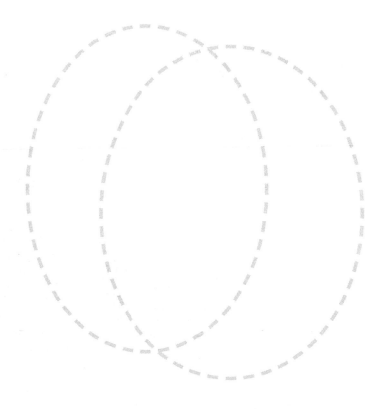

Down Dog

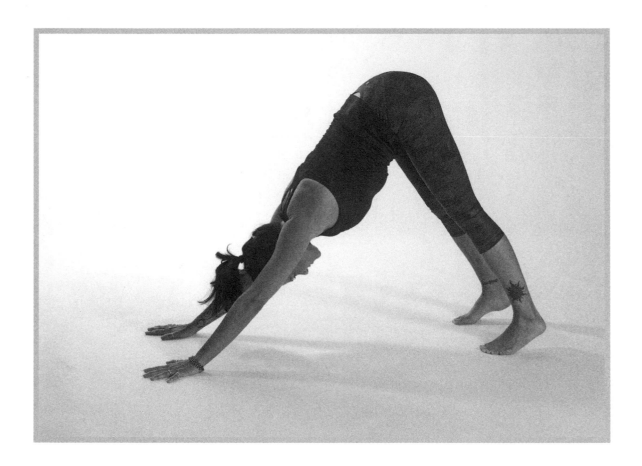

From Plank pose, keep your hands shoulder-width apart with palms flat and fingers spread, place your feet hip-width to shoulders-width apart, lift your tailbone to the sky, and create an upside-down "V" shape with your body. Keep the back flat and sink into the hamstring stretch. If your hamstrings are tight, then it is more important to keep the back flat and start with bent knees.

Variations of Down Dog

Down Dog Kicks

Starting in Down Dog, kick the right leg up to the sky and bring it back down to Down Dog. Repeat on the other side.

Shooting Star

Assuming the Down Dog position, sink the weight into the left foot and heel and raise the right leg to the sky, keeping the hips square while pushing the floor away with your hands. Repeat on the other side.

Shooting Star in Motion

rom Shooting Star pose, with your right leg up to the sky, bend the right knee and at the same time start to twist the torso open and peek under your right armpit up to the sky. Stay there and continue to twist until you flip the body completely open, dropping your right leg to the floor on the other side of your left leg with your chest facing the ceiling.

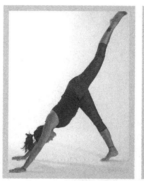
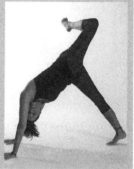
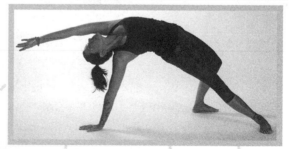

Downward Dog Push-Ups

Starting in Downward Dog, bend the elbows out to the side and let the head descend down as close to touching the floor as you can, keeping the hands flat and fingers spread. Push the arms straight again and repeat.

Plow

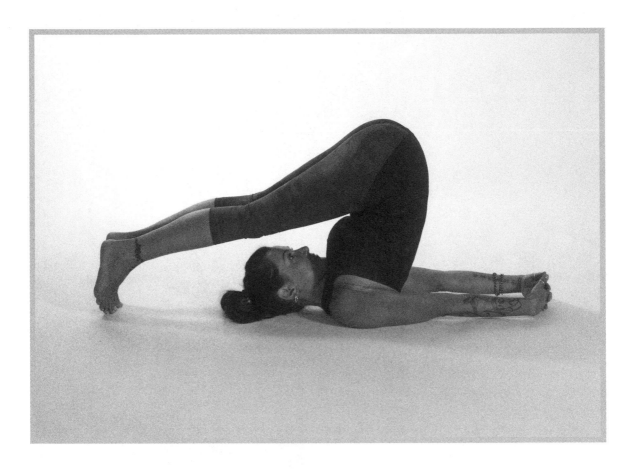

Lying down on your back, draw the knees into your chest. Press the arms down into the floor alongside your body with palms facing down. Press firmly into the arms and bring the legs over your head. If you are flexible enough, the toes will touch the floor behind your head and you can snuggle the shoulder blades under to protect the neck and interlace your fingers, extending your arms along the floor. If you are not flexible enough, still snuggle the shoulder blades under, but instead bend the elbows and place your hands, with palms flat, on your lower back for support. Both levels should be deep enough to feel the stretch of the back body, but still be able to breathe. Straighten the legs as much as you can and hold.

Variations of Plow

Plow Pedal

In Plow position, bend the elbows and place the palms flat on your back. With the legs over the face and parallel to the floor, start a pedaling action with the legs for the suggested amount of time.

Shoulder Stand

From Plow pose, bend the elbows and place the palms flat on your back. Snuggle the shoulders under and straighten the legs up to the sky. You should feel as though the upper arms are pressing down into the floor, with the hands pressing into the back and pushing the body up. Try to bring the chest as close to the chin as possible.

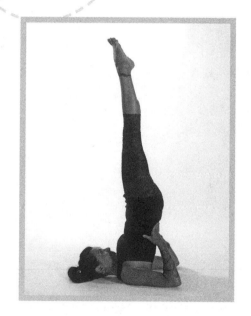

Heavy Legs

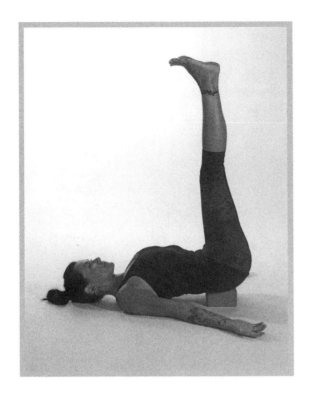 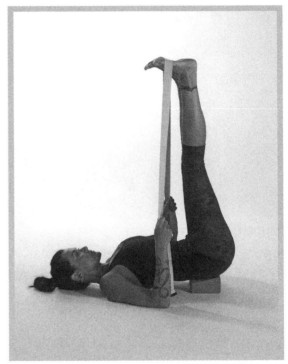

Lying on your back, bend the knees with the feet flat on the floor. Raise the hips and place a yoga block under the lower hips. Straighten the legs up to the sky and hold.

To make this pose most enjoyable, use a yoga strap across the feet, holding each side of the strap in the appropriate hand.

Searchlights

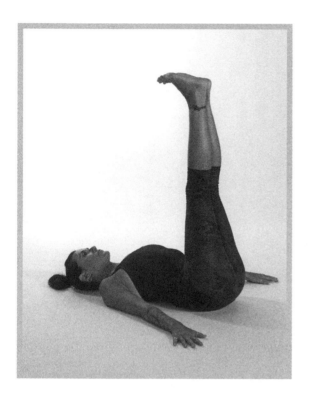 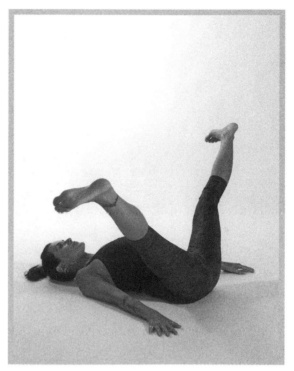

In Heavy Legs positioning, open the legs wide into a straddle position and then bring them together, repeat.

Handstand

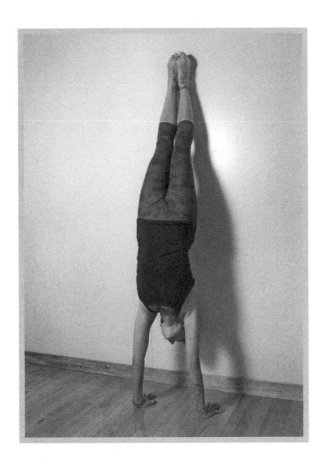

Place your hands on the floor a foot away from a sturdy wall. Your hands should be shoulder-width apart with palms flat and fingers spread. Lift one leg up and kick to the wall. Push the floor away and firm up the arms, rest your legs against the wall, and hold.

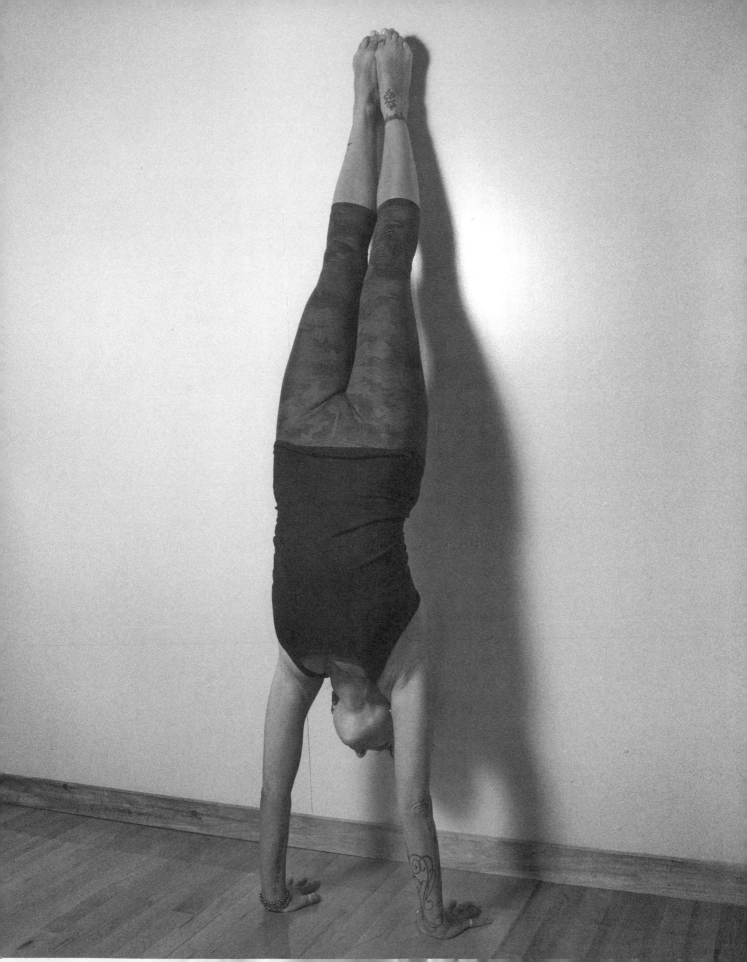

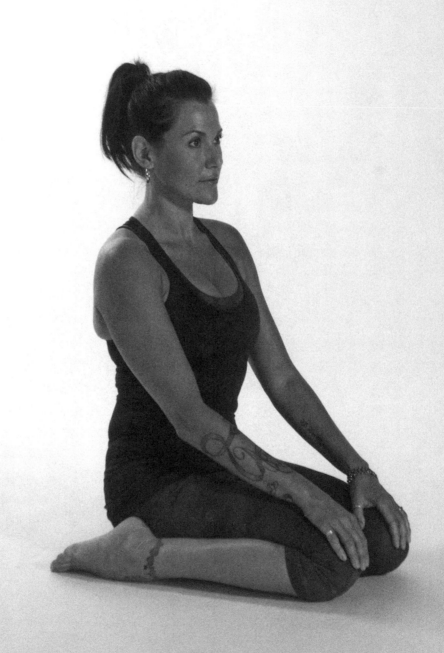

Seated Poses

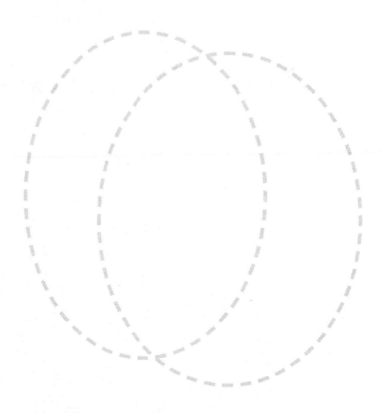

Boat

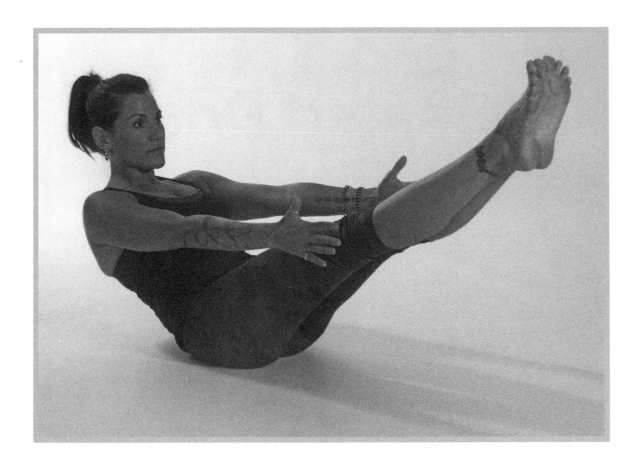

Lean back on your butt in a seated position. Extend the arms toward the front of the room, keeping the arms parallel to the floor. Straighten the legs so the toes are in alignment with your view point. Be sure to keep the back as straight as you can, engage the abdominals, and hold.

Variations of Boat

Boat-Ins

Starting from Boat position, gradually draw the knees into your chest, pause, and then extend them back out again. Repeat.

Boat–Ins Alternate Legs

Perform Boat-Ins and alternate legs.

Boat Twists

Holding Boat pose, interlace your fingers. While maintaining the integrity of Boat, bring the hands to the floor on the outside of the left hip, and switch. Be careful and precise throughout these movements. For an extra challenge, you can perform this movement using a medicine ball.

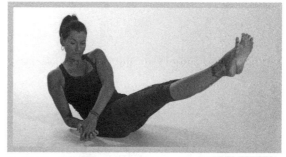

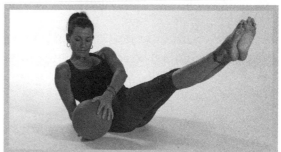

Seated Mountain

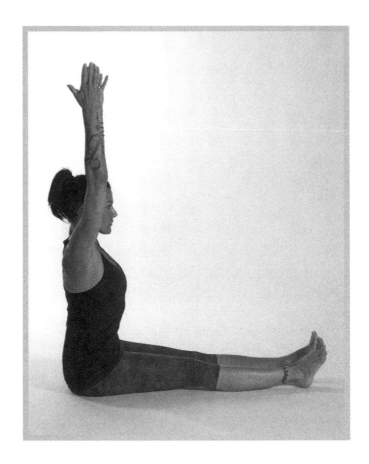

Come to a natural seated position, sitting upright on the sit bones with the spine tall and long, legs extended straight out in front of you, and toes facing up. Keep the legs energized and let the arms fall down by your side or extend the arms straight up to the sky with palms facing each other.

Variations of Seated Mountain

Extended Leg Seated Twist

In Seated Mountain Pose, hold the arms out to the sides, bend the elbows 90 degrees and twist deeply to the left and then deeply to the right.

Seated Forward Bend

Follow the same technique as the Seated Mountain pose, but fold over from the hips as far as you can with a straight and flat back.

Hikers

Start in Seated Mountain pose with the arms extended up to the sky and the upper arms alongside the head. Maintain a tall and strong back and lift the right leg an inch off the floor. Pause and switch to the other side.

Kaleidoscopes

Start in Seated Mountain pose with the arms extended up to the sky. Place your heels on sliders then slide open the legs into a straddle position and slide them back again. Repeat.

Wobbles

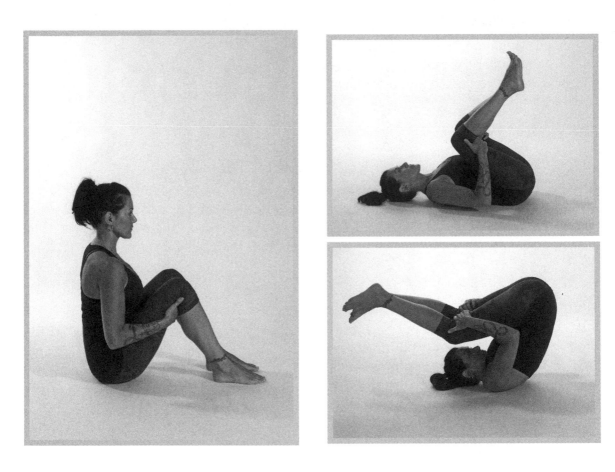

Lying on your back, draw your knees into your chest and wrap your arms around the back of your thighs and simply rock and roll on your back like you did when you were a child.

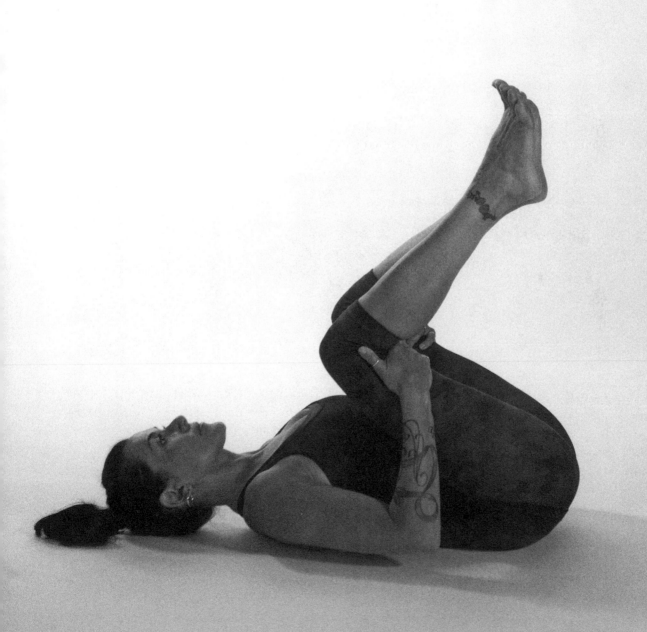

Half Hero

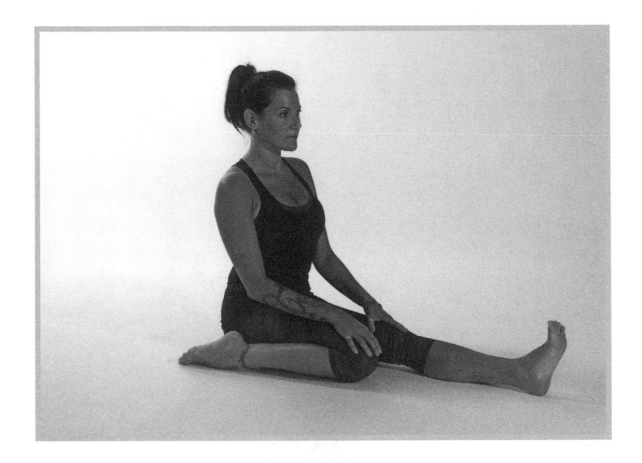

Sitting on the floor, extend the right leg long and fold the left knee so the left foot is alongside the left hip. Ultimately you should be sitting on the floor with both butt cheeks firm to the ground. If you are not ready for this, sit on a rolled-up towel or yoga block until you are flexible enough to sit on the floor. A word of caution: This is a safe pose for the knees, however, you should always see the bottom of the foot facing straight up to the sky to protect the knee and keep the knee in a natural flexion. Repeat on the other side.

Variation of Half Hero

Hero

Follow the same positioning as Half Hero, but with both knees bent. If you have trouble with this, start with these suggestions: Use a rolled-up towel behind the knees to alleviate any knee pain. If that is okay then you can sit back on the heels. The next step is to separate the feet and sit on a yoga block between the feet until you are flexible enough to sit on the floor between your feet in full expression of Hero pose.

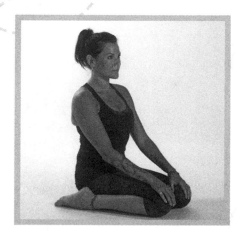

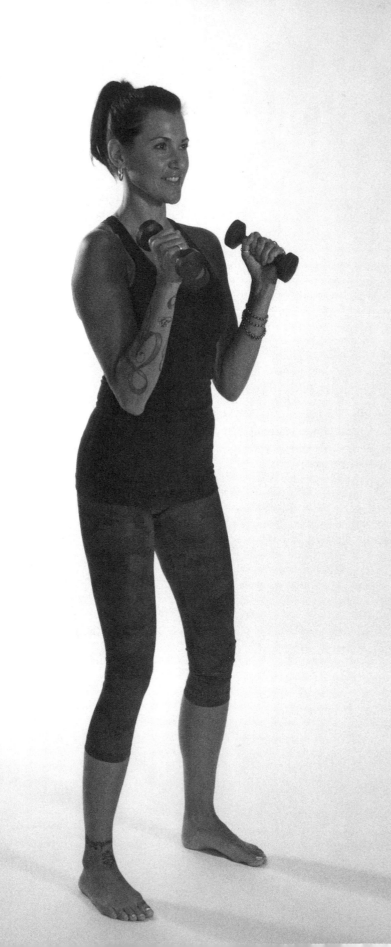

Weightlifting Moves

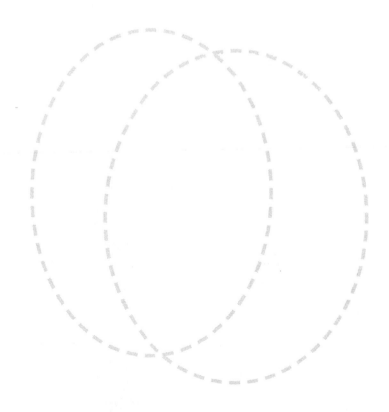

Chest Press

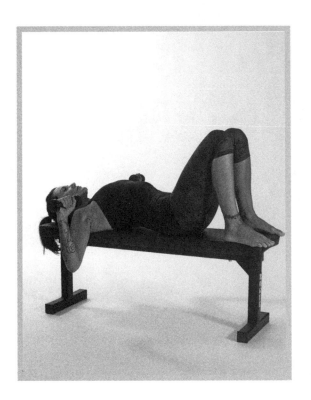 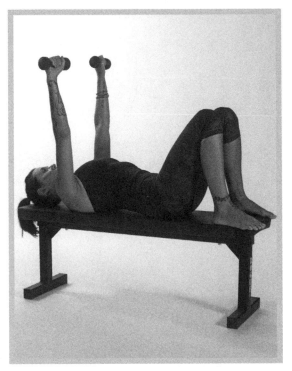

Lie on the bench with a dumbbell in each hand and your feet flat on the floor, or place your feet up on the bench if it's more comfortable. Push the dumbbells up so that your arms are directly over your shoulders and your palms are facing up. Lower the dumbbells back down until your elbows are slightly below your shoulders. Roll your shoulder blades back and push the weights back up, taking care not to lock your elbows or allow your shoulder blades to rise off the bench.

Chest Fly

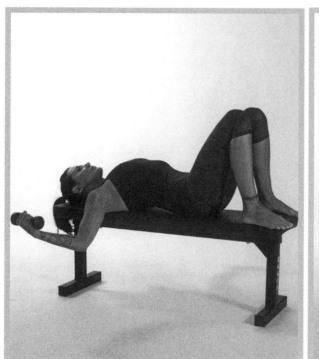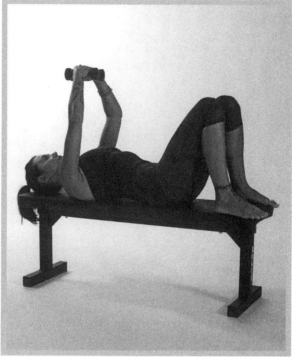

Lying on the bench with a dumbbell in each hand, look directly up at the ceiling, keeping your spine in alignment. As you inhale, slowly extend your elbows out to the side. You should be making a "T" with your upper body, with the elbows slightly bent. Exhale as you carefully bring the dumbbells together over the center of your chest, as though you are hugging a barrel. Once the dumbbells come together, slowly bring them back to their starting position. Keep the back flat on the bench the entire time.

Triceps Cross Face

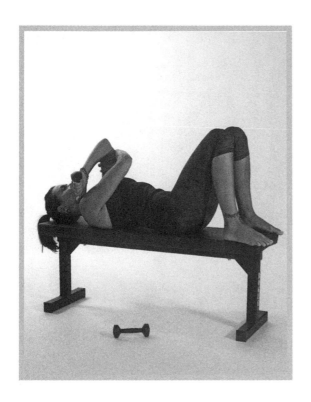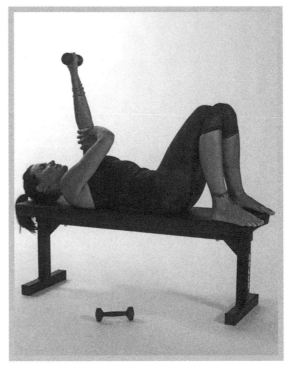

Lie down on your back on the floor or bench with a weight in your right hand. Straighten the right arm up to the sky directly from your shoulder, with the palm facing forward. Take your left hand and firmly grab your right arm below the elbow to stabilize the right arm position. Hinge the right elbow, carefully lowering the weight next to the left ear and return. Repeat on the other side.

Rows

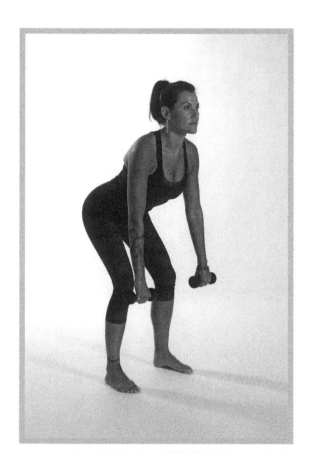 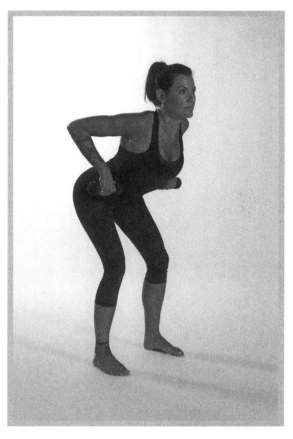

Bend the knees slightly and bend over, keeping the back straight. Grasp dumbbells with an overhand grip. Pull the weights to your upper waist. Straighten the arms until the arms are extended and the shoulders are stretched downward. Repeat.

Shoulder Press

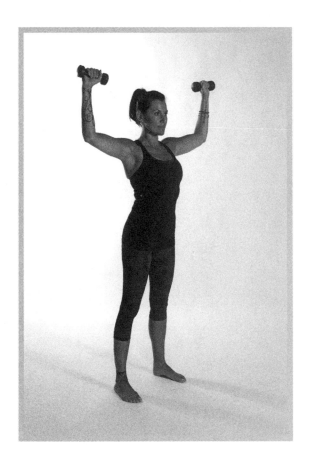 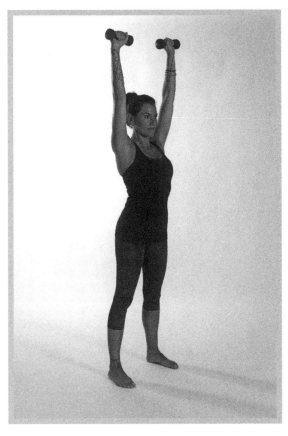

Hold a dumbbell in each hand and stand with your back straight and tall. Plant your feet firmly on the floor. Bend your elbows and raise your upper arms to shoulder height so the dumbbells are at ear level and the elbows form a 90-degree angle. Push the dumbbells up and in until the ends of the dumbbells touch lightly, directly over your head, and then lower the dumbbells back to ear level. Repeat.

Front Shoulder Raise

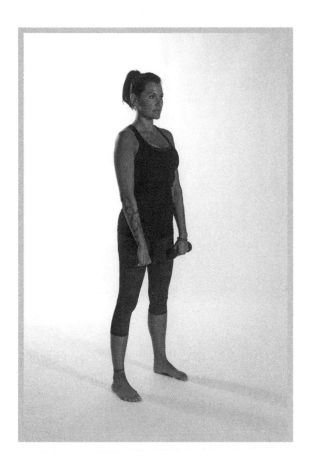 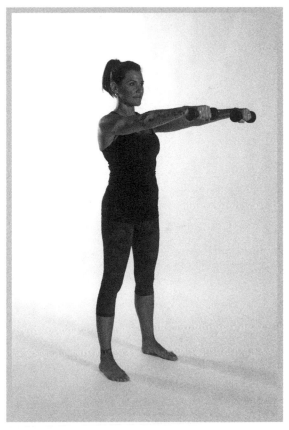

Holding a dumbbell in each hand, position the arms in front of your body with palms facing the floor. Keeping the shoulders down, raise the arms straight out in front of you until the arms are shoulder height, then return them to the starting position.

Biceps Curl

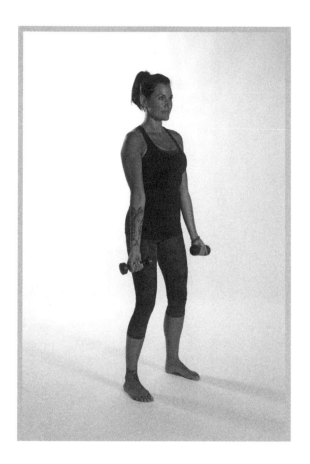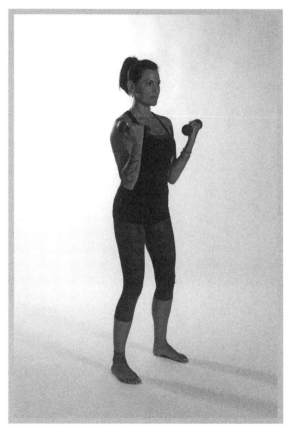

Hold a dumbbell in each hand and stand with your feet hips-width apart. Let your arms hang down at your sides with your palms forward. Firm up your core and stand tall, keeping your knees slightly bent. Curl both arms upward until they're in front of your shoulders, with the palms facing your shoulders. Slowly lower the dumbbells back down and repeat.

Hammer Curl

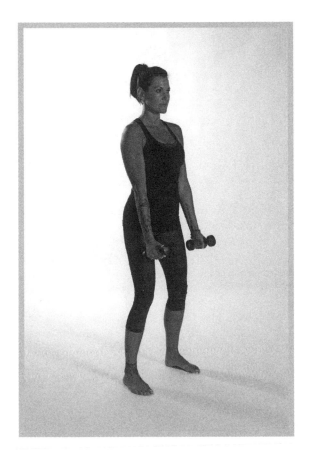 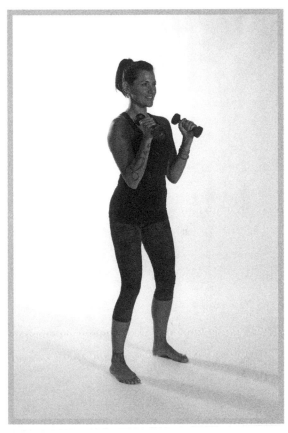

Hold a dumbbell in each hand. Grip the dumbbells and rotate the hands so the palms are facing each other. When you curl with this grip, your thumb will lead the motion of each hand. Curl one of the dumbbells upward by contracting the biceps muscle. Avoid movement in the upper arm and shoulder joint. Slowly lower the dumbbell to the starting position and then repeat with the alternate hand.

Dead Lift

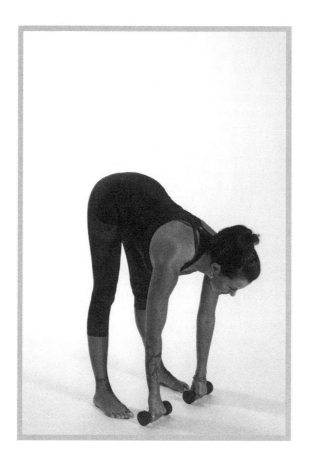 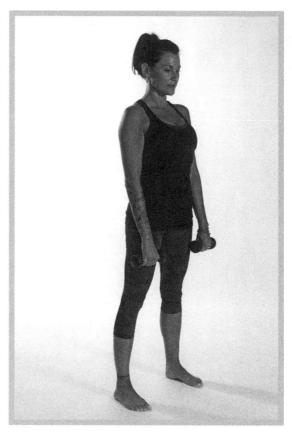

Stand with the bar or dumbbells above the center of your feet, with the feet hips-width or shoulders-width apart. Grab the bar over the top with palms facing down so that your arms are vertical to the floor. Bend through your knees until your shins hit the bar, which must remain above the middle of your feet. Lift your chest, keeping your head in line with the rest of your spine. Standing up, pull the bar or dumbbells, keeping the bar close to your body, and roll it over your knees and thighs until your hips and knees are locked. Do not lean back at the top. Return, repeat.

Double Arm Swing

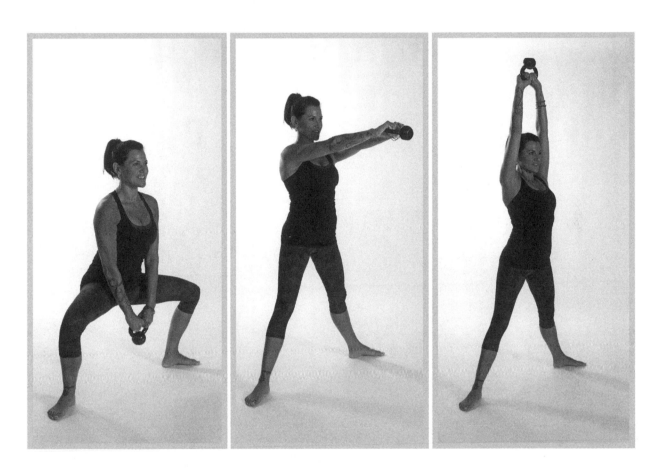

Straddle a kettlebell with your feet slightly wider than shoulder-width apart. Squat down with the arms extended downward between your legs and grab the kettlebell with both hands using an overhand grip.

Pull the kettlebell up and forward off the floor by standing up. Immediately squat down slightly and swing the kettlebell back under the hips. Swing the kettlebell up by raising the upper body upright and extending the legs. Continue to swing the kettlebell back down between the legs and up higher on each swing until the highest point reaches just above your head.

Swing the kettlebell back down between your legs. Allow the kettlebell to swing forward, but do not extend your hips and knees. Slow the kettlebell's swing and place it on the floor between your feet to return to a Dead Lift posture.

Triceps Extension

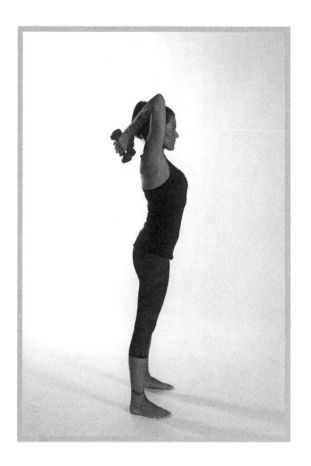 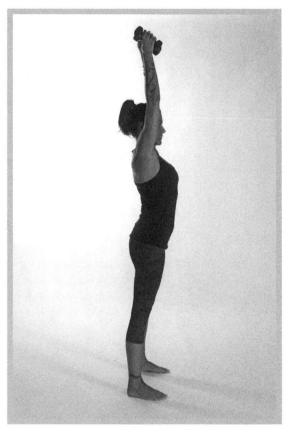

Stand with a dumbbell held in each hand. With your feet about shoulder-width apart, lift the dumbbells over your head until both arms are fully extended toward the ceiling. The palms of the hands should be facing each other. Keeping your upper arms close to your head with your elbows in and arms perpendicular to the floor, hinge the elbows and lower the weights behind your head until your forearms touch your biceps. The upper arms should remain stationary and only the forearms should move. Return to the starting extended position and repeat.

Calf Raise Trio

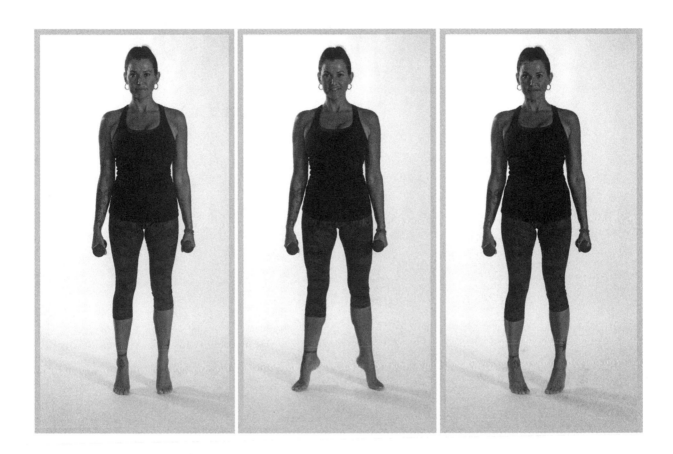

Stand with feet hips-width apart and parallel. Holding a dumbbell in each hand, push into the toes and lift the heels as far off the floor as possible, then lower the heels and repeat. Next, turn the feet out to 45-degree angles and do the same movement, repeating for the desired amount of time. Finally, pigeon toe the feet and raise and lower the heels.

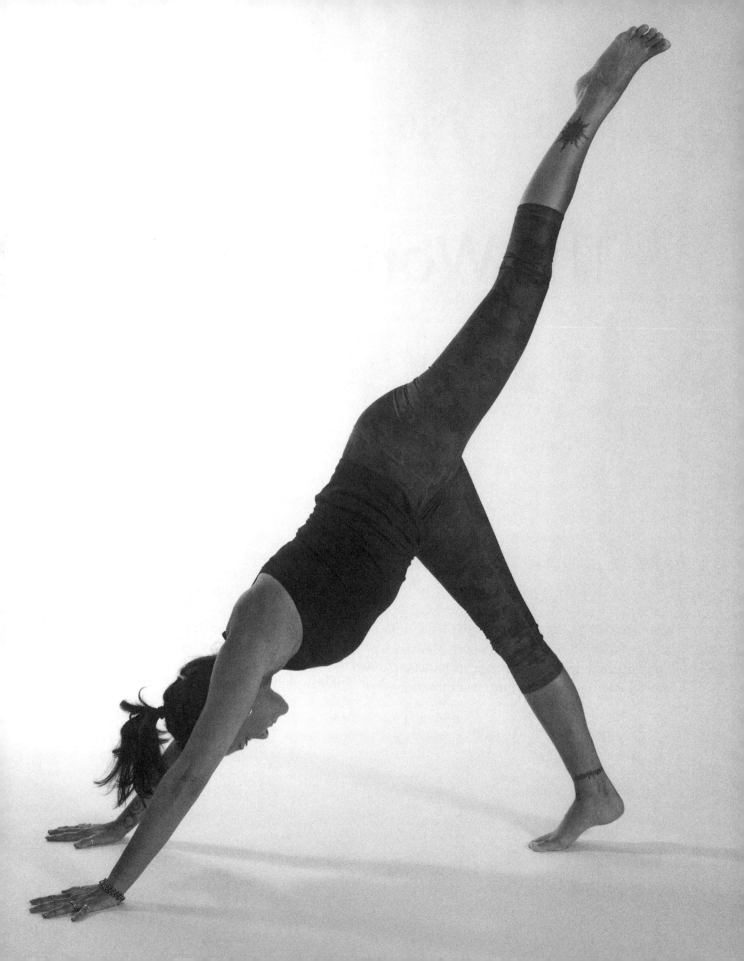

The **Workouts**   8

These workouts are designed to be user-friendly and customizable to *your* body and *your* fitness goals. The workouts are arranged into three levels—Beginner, Intermediate, and Advanced—with six weeks of workouts for each level.

You will work out four days each week (we recommend Monday, Wednesday, Friday, and Saturday with days of rest in between) and for each day you will find clear directions on when and how to perform the workouts.

Pick your level of fitness and follow the guide. (Refer to the Index of Exercises on page 183 to locate each exercise.)

The duration of the workouts is completely determined by you and should be based on the goals you have set for yourself. The workouts are set up as a continuous flow, and at the end of the flow (depending on your energy level and time constraints) you will repeat the flow one to three more times.

As you become more adept at the workouts, you can choose to add additional weights to increase resistance, build more muscle, and increase your heart rate. You can start by adding ½ to 1-pound wrist and/or ankle weights. Later on, you may also want to add a 10-15 pound weighted vest.

These workouts are designed for each exercise to move seamlessly into the next in a smooth, yoga-inspired way. Before you start, review the moves first and visualize how your body will move through the poses. You may also find it helpful to prop up the book in front of you to avoid having to walk back and forth to note the next move. Also, make sure to set up your equipment for each workout before you begin so that you can keep the flow constant.

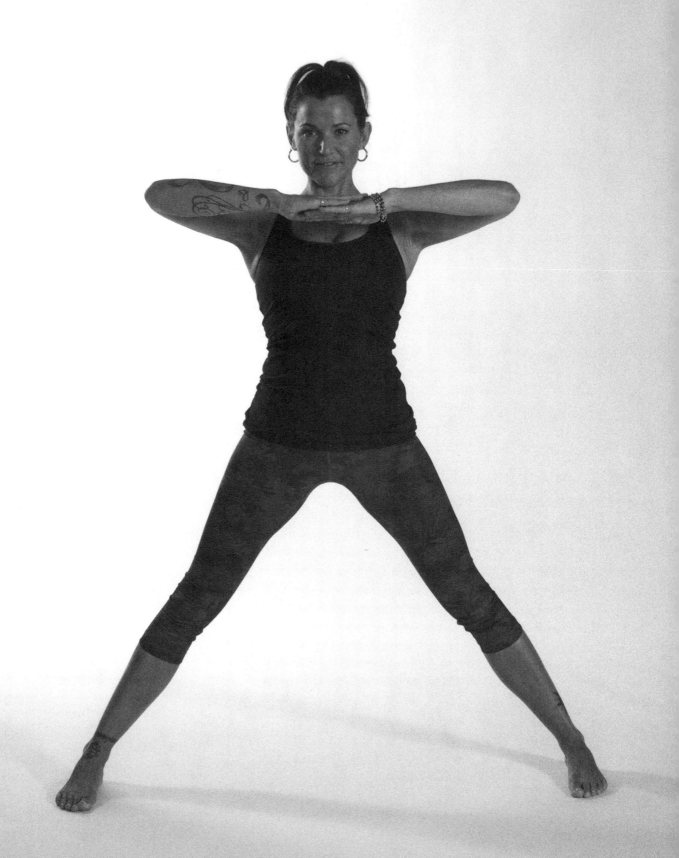

Beginner
Workouts

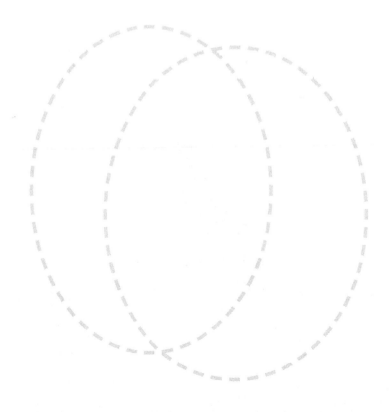

BEGINNER WORKOUT: WEEK 1	
Day 1 & 3	**Day 2 & 4**
Warm-Up	**Warm-Up**
Chateranga—Upward Dog—Down Dog—Plank—Table	Standing Forward Bend—Plank—Chateranga—Upward Dog—Down Dog
3-Legged Table: Lift the right leg and extend back. Lift the left leg and extend back. Pulse 10 times on each side, 3 sets each side	Right foot forward, Crescent—Crescent Lunge Twist
Table—High Knees—Folding Table-Crossovers: 10 reps each on both legs	Crescent—Half Hero—Crescent—Warrior 3: 3 sets
Side Plank—Plank—Side Plank—Plank: 3 sets	Standing Forward Bend
Table Scissors: 10 reps each leg, 3 sets	Left foot forward, Crescent—Crescent Lunge Twist
Half Side Plank with Karate Kick: 10 reps each leg	Crescent—Half Hero—Crescent—Warrior 3: 3 sets
Do the whole routine 1-3+ times	Standing Forward Bend
Pick 3 long, deep holds	Camel: 20 seconds Camel Praise: 5 reps Quad Crunch: 5 reps Plank—Chateranga to belly—3 push-ups (knees down if needed) Bow: 5 seconds Cobra—Cobra Push-Up: 5 reps Down Dog
	Child's Pose
	Do the whole routine 1-3+ times
	Pick 3 long, deep holds
NOTES:	

BEGINNER WORKOUT: WEEK 2	
Day 1 & 3	**Day 2 & 4**
Warm-Up	**Warm-Up**
Standing Forward Bend—Plank—Chateranga—Upward Dog—Down Dog	Standing Forward Bend—Plank—Chateranga—Upward Dog—Down Dog
Crescent Lunge (right foot forward)—Plank—Chateranga—Upward Dog—Down Dog: 3 reps	Crescent Lunge (right leg forward)—Crescent Lunge Twist—Crescent Lunge
Crescent Lunge (left foot forward)—Plank—Chateranga—Upward Dog—Down Dog: 3 reps	Hold the Bundle (left knee to chest)—Crescent Lunge: 3 reps
Crescent Lunge (right foot forward)—SOS (10 reps)—Crescent Lunge Twist (hold 5 seconds)	Standing Forward Bend: hold 10 seconds
Crescent Lunge (left foot forward)—SOS (10 reps)—Crescent Lunge Twist (hold 5 seconds)	Crescent Lunge (left leg forward)—Crescent Lunge Twist—Crescent Lunge
Straddle Forward Bend: hold 5 seconds Triangle (right side)—Revolving Triangle Triangle (left side)—Revolving Triangle Right Angle (right side)—Fan the Fire: 5 reps Right Angle (left side)—Fan the Fire: 5 reps	Hold the Bundle (right knee to chest)—Crescent Lunge: 3 reps
	Standing Forward Bend: hold 10 seconds
Do the whole routine 1-3+ times	Plank—Down Dog Crescent Lunge (right foot forward) Dragonfly: 10 seconds Plank Crescent Lunge (left foot forward) Dragonfly: 10 seconds Plank Standing Forward Bend—Squat—Rockets: 3 reps
Pick 3 long, deep holds	Wobbles (seated): 3 reps Plow—Shoulder Stand—Heavy Legs—Chest Press: 5 reps Chest Fly: 5 reps Triceps Cross Face: 5 reps
	Do the whole routine 1-3+ times
	Pick 3 long, deep holds
NOTES:	

BEGINNER WORKOUT: WEEK 3	
Day 1 & 3	**Day 2 & 4**
Warm-Up Standing Forward Bend—Halfway-Up Flat Back: hold 5 seconds Double Arm Row: 5 reps Repeat for 3 sets Plank—Chateranga—Upward Dog—Down Dog Half Side Squat (right foot forward) Back and forth 3 reps each side Turn to the front Crescent Lunge: 5 seconds Crescent Lunge Twist: 5 seconds Plank—Chateranga—Upward Dog—Down Dog Half Side Squat (left foot forward) Back and forth 3 reps each side Turn to the front Crescent Lunge: 5 seconds Crescent Lunge Twist: 5 seconds Plank—Chateranga—Upward Dog—Down Dog Squat: hold 30 seconds Wobbles: 5 Reps Inverted Plank (seated): 5 reps Boat (hold 5 seconds)—Boat-Ins (10 reps) Wobbles: 5 reps Inverted Plank (seated): 5 reps Boat-Ins Alternate Legs: 5 reps each side Seated Mountain (arms extended): hold 5 seconds Hikers: 10 reps each side Seated Forward Bend: hold 1 minute **Do the whole routine 1-3+ times** **Pick 3 long, deep holds**	**Warm-Up** Plank—Chateranga—Upward Dog—Down Dog (hold 10 seconds) Down Dog Kicks: 10 reps each side Standing Forward Bend—Chair (hold 30 seconds)—Standing Forward Bend Repeat 3 sets Chair Chair Twist (right)—Chair—Chair Twist (left)—Chair Repeat Chair Twist (right)—Lunge Twist (right): hold 5 seconds Unwind the body into Triangle (right)—Triangle Flags (hold 5 seconds) Runner's Lunge—Knee Kissers (5 reps)—On Your Marks (5 reps) Plank—Chateranga—Upward Dog—Down Dog (hold 10 seconds) Standing Forward Bend Chair Repeat on the other side Plank—Wrench: 2 times each side Plank—Forearm Plank—Plank—Forearm Plank (hold 30 seconds) **Do the whole routine 1-3+ times** **Pick 3 long, deep holds**
NOTES:	

BEGINNER WORKOUT: WEEK 4	
Day 1 & 3	**Day 2 & 4**
Warm-Up	**Warm-Up**
Down Dog—Shooting Star—Shooting Star in Motion—Plank—Knee Kisser—Shooting Star—Shooting Star in Motion—Plank—Knee Kisser Plank—Chateranga—Upward Dog—Down Dog Repeat on the other side	Standing Forward Bend (hold 10 seconds)—Plank Wrench: 2 reps each side (knees down) Chateranga—Upward Dog—Down Dog—Plank—push-ups (knees down), 10 reps
Down Dog—Warrior 2 (right leg forward): hold 30 seconds Biceps Curl in Warrior 2 (no weights): 10 reps Shoulder Press in Warrior 2 (no weights): 10 reps Reverse Warrior (hold 30 seconds)—Warrior 2 (hold 30 seconds) Right Angle (hold 30 seconds)—Fan the Fire: 5 reps (left arm) Reverse Warrior (hold 30 seconds)—Right Angle (hold 30 seconds)—Fan the Fire: 5 Reps in opposite direction Warrior 1—Biceps Curl: 5 reps	Lower to belly Locust—lower to belly: 5 reps Canoes: 10 reps Child's Pose—Boat (hold 10 seconds)—Boat-Ins (10 reps)—Boat Twist (10 reps) Inverted Plank (hold 10 seconds)—Shark Attack (10 reps) Roll over legs to Standing Forward Bend (10 reps)—Standing Mountain—Serpentine Jump (10 reps) Run in place 30 seconds—Standing Forward Bend—Plank—Knee Kissers (5 reps each side)
Crescent Lunge (hold 30 seconds)—Warrior 3—Crescent Lunge—Pinwheels (30 seconds) Warrior 3—Hold the Bundle (left knee in)—Deliver the Bundle: 5 reps	Chateranga—Cobra—Cobra Push-Ups (10 reps)—Down Dog—Down Dog Push-Ups (10 reps) **Do the whole routine 1-3+ times** **Pick 3 long, deep holds**
Standing Mountain—Plank—Chateranga—Upward Dog—Down Dog Plank—Chateranga—Upward Dog—Down Dog Repeat on the other side, left foot forward **Do the whole routine 1-3+ times** **Pick 3 long, deep holds**	
NOTES:	

BEGINNER WORKOUT: WEEK 5	
Day 1 & 3	**Day 2 & 4**
Warm-Up Chateranga—Upward Dog—Down Dog (hold 30 seconds) Bring the right leg up—Shooting Star—Runner's Lunge (right foot forward)—Pinwheels (30 seconds)—Stop Traffic (hold 30 seconds) Eagle Lunge (hold 30 seconds)—Eagle—Eagle Lunge—Eagle—Eagle Lunge—Eagle Crescent Lunge—Crescent Lunge Twist (hold 30 seconds) Release Plank (hold 30 seconds)—Half Side Plank—5 top arm circles—Half Side Plank with Karate Kick (5 reps) Plank—Chateranga—Plank—Chateranga—Upward Dog—Down Dog Repeat on other side **Do the whole routine 1-3+ times** **Pick 3 long, deep holds**	**Warm-Up** Child's Pose—Slither—Cobra—Cobra Push-Ups (5 reps)—Slither—Child's Pose Repeat 3 sets Down Dog—Shooting Star (right leg) Shooting Star (left leg) Table—Seated Mountain—Extended Leg Seated Twist (30 seconds)—Stop Traffic (30 seconds) Hikers (3 reps each side)—Plow—Plow Pedal (20 each leg) Wobbles (5 reps)—Seated Forward Bend—Kaleidoscopes (10 reps) Bridge—Bridge Lifts (10 reps)—Camel (hold 30 seconds)—Hero (hold 1 minute) **Do the whole routine 1-3+ times** **Pick 3 long, deep holds**
NOTES:	

| BEGINNER WORKOUT: WEEK 6 ||
Day 1 & 3	Day 2 & 4
Warm-Up	**Warm-Up**
Chateranga—Upward Dog—Down Dog Crescent Lunge (right foot forward)—Crescent Twist—Crescent Lunge Hammie Curl (3 reps)	Run in place 2 minutes Wall Squat: 30 seconds Toe Balance Squat—Standing Forward Bend: 10 sets Wobbles: 5 reps Twisted Root Abdominals: 10 reps each side
Sit back to Half Hero—Crescent: 5 sets	
Crescent Lunge—Warrior 3—Crescent Lunge: 3 sets End in Warrior 3—Standing Split (left leg up)—Split Kicks (5 reps each side) Roll to Mountain Pose—Standing Back-bend—Standing Forward Bend Grab barbell Deadlift: 10 reps Roll to stand with barbell Calf Raise Trio: 10 reps each position Cross-Kicks: 1 minute Side-to-Side Chair: 1 minute Standing Forward Bend—Split Kicks (5 reps each leg)—Plank—Chateranga—Upward Dog—Down Dog	Wobbles (5 reps)—Standing Forward Bend—Plank—Chateranga—Upward Dog—Down Dog Down Dog Push-Ups: 10 reps Plank: hold 30 seconds Forearm Plank—Plank—Forearm Plank: 5 sets Forearm Plank: hold 30 seconds Plank—Mountain Climbers (30 seconds) Push-ups (knees down): 5 reps Plank—Down Dog—Down Dog Push-Ups (5 reps) Standing Forward Bend—Standing Mountain Step-Ups (5 reps each leg)—Standing Mountain
Repeat on other side from the top	
Do the whole routine 1-3+ times	Figure 4 Chair (left foot across)—Figure 4 Chair Fold (5 reps) Skaters (left leg back): 5 reps Figure 4 Chair (right foot across)—Figure 4 Chair Folds (5 reps) Skaters (right leg back): 5 reps Standing Forward Bend
Pick 3 long, deep holds	
	Do the whole routine 1-3+ times
	Pick 3 long, deep holds
NOTES:	

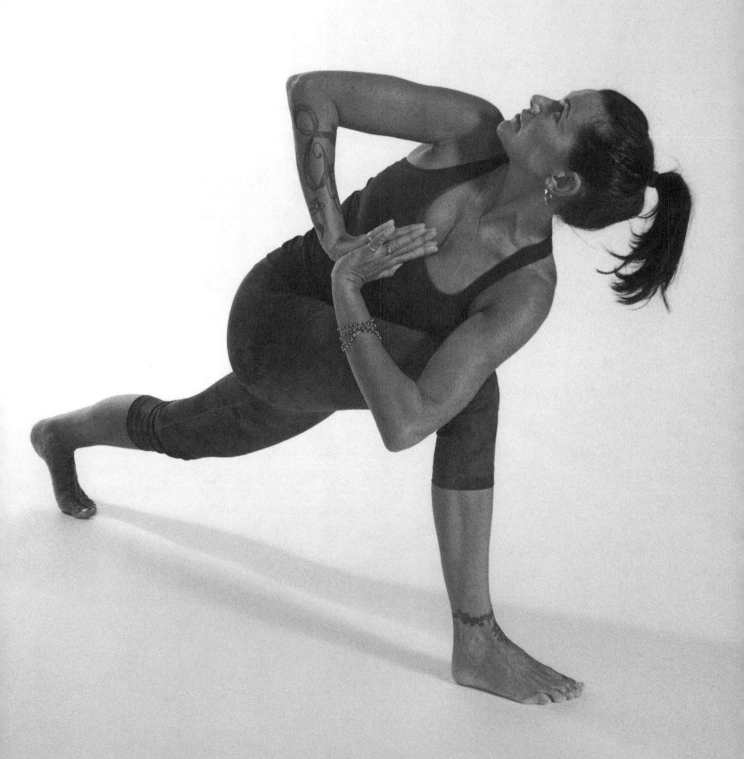

Intermediate Workouts

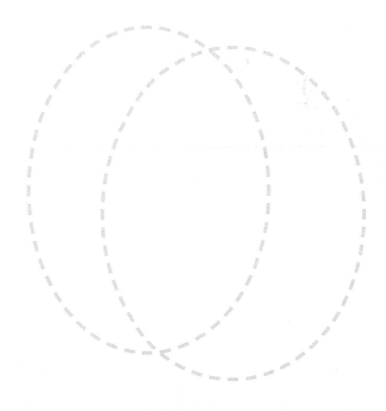

INTERMEDIATE WORKOUT: WEEK 1	
Day 1 & 3	**Day 2 & 4**
Warm-Up Chateranga—Upward Dog—Down Dog Plank—Heel Drops (10 reps each side)— Knee to Nose (5 reps each side) Plank—Table Scissor (right leg): 5 reps Plank—Table Scissor (left leg): 5 reps Plank Cross-Over (right leg): 5 reps Plank Cross-Over (left leg): 5 reps Side Plank (right)—Plank—Chateranga— Plank—Side Plank (left)—Plank: 3 sets Plank: hold 1 minute Mountain Climbers: 1 minute Faux Jump Rope: 30 seconds High Knees: 30 seconds Butt Kicks: 30 seconds **Do the whole routine 1-3+ times** **Pick 3 long, deep holds**	**Warm-Up** Standing Forward Bend—Plank—Chater- anga—Upward Dog—Down Dog: 3 sets Warrior 1 (right foot forward): hold 30 sec- onds Runner's Lunge—Lunge Twist (hold 30 seconds) Runner's Lunge—Half Hero—Warrior 1— Warrior 3: 5 sets Standing Forward Bend Repeat on the other side Standing Forward Bend—Table—Camel (hold 30 seconds) Camel Praise: 15 reps Quad Crunch: 15 reps Plank—Chateranga—Bow (hold 30 sec- onds) Cobra—Cobra Push-Ups (10 reps)—Down Dog (hold 30 seconds)—Child's Pose **Do the whole routine 1-3+ times** **Pick 3 long, deep holds**
NOTES:	

INTERMEDIATE WORKOUT: WEEK 2	
Day 1 & 3	**Day 2 & 4**
Warm-Up Standing Forward Bend—Plank—Chateranga—Upward Dog—Down Dog Runner's Lunge (right foot forward)—On Your Marks (10 reps) Chateranga—Upward Dog—Down Dog—Runner's Lunge (left foot forward)—On Your Marks (10 reps) Do 3 sets each side Runner's Lunge (right foot forward)—SOS (15 reps)—Pinwheels (15 reps) Lunge Twist: hold 30 seconds Repeat on other side Standing Straddle Forward Bend Genies: 30 seconds Standing Straddle Forward Bend: hold 30 seconds Triangle (right, hold 30 seconds)—Triangle Flags (hold 30 seconds)—Revolving Triangle (hold 30 seconds) Standing Straddle Forward Bend—Triangle (left, hold 30 seconds)—Triangle Flags (hold 30 seconds)—Revolving Triangle (hold 30 seconds) Standing Mountain (at the front of the mat)—Plank—Chateranga—Upward Dog—Down Dog Right Angle (right foot forward, hold 30 seconds)—Right Angle Flag (hold 30 seconds)—Plank—Standing Mountain—Cross-Kicks (30 seconds) Yoga Burpees: 3 sets Right Angle (left foot forward, hold 30 seconds)—Right Angle Flag (hold 30 seconds)—Plank—Standing Mountain—Cross-Kicks (30 seconds) **Do the whole routine 1-3+ times** **Pick 3 long, deep holds**	**Warm-Up** Standing Forward Bend—Plank—Chateranga—Upward Dog—Down Dog Crescent Lunge (right foot forward)—Pinwheels (30 seconds) Crescent Lunge—Hold the Bundle (holding left leg)—Deliver the Bundle (5 reps) Crescent Lunge: 3 sets Standing Forward Bend Repeat on the other side Lunge (right foot forward)—Dragonfly (hold 30 seconds) Plank: hold 30 seconds Repeat other side Plank—Squat (hold 30 seconds)—Rockets (10 reps)—Take-Offs (10 reps) Wobbles (5 reps)—Plow (hold 30 seconds)—Plow Pedal (1 minute)—Shoulder Stand (hold 1 minute)—Heavy Legs—Chest Press (10 reps while in Heavy Legs) Chest Fly: 10 reps Put your feet down Triceps Cross Face: 10 reps each side Searchlights: 10 reps Seals: 1 minute **Do the whole routine 1-3+ times** **Pick 3 long, deep holds**
NOTES:	

INTERMEDIATE WORKOUT: WEEK 3	
Day 1 & 3	**Day 2 & 4**
Warm-Up Standing Forward Bend—Squats (with weights, 20 reps) Standing Mountain—Side to Side Chair (1 minute) Double Arm Row: 10 reps Repeat 3 sets Plank—Chateranga—Upward Dog—Down Dog Half Side Squat (right foot forward, arms up for increased difficulty) Half Side Squat (left foot forward) 3 reps each side Crescent Lunge (right foot forward): hold 30 seconds Crescent Twist (hold 30 seconds) Plank—Chateranga—Upward Dog—Down Dog Half Side Squat (right foot forward, arms up for increased difficulty) Half Side Squat (left foot forward) 3 reps each side Crescent Lunge (left foot forward): hold 30 seconds Crescent Twist: hold 30 seconds Plank—Squat—Rockets (20 reps weighted) Wobbles: 5 reps Inverted Plank (5 reps)—Boat (hold 30 seconds)—Boat-Ins (10 reps) Wobbles: 5 reps Inverted Plank (hold 30 seconds) Rockettes: 5 reps each side Hikers (10 reps each leg holding arms over head with light weights) Seated Forward Bend: hold 1 minute **Do the whole routine 1-3+ times** **Pick 3 long, deep holds**	**Warm-Up** Standing Forward Bend: hold 1 minute with sandbag across forearms Plank—Chateranga—Upward Dog—Down Dog (hold 1 minute) Standing Forward Bend—Split Kicks (10 reps each side) Standing Forward Bend—Double Arm Swing (5 reps) Chair: hold 30 seconds Standing Forward Bend Repeat 3 sets (while holding a smaller kettlebell the whole time, even when arms extended in Chair) Release kettlebell Chair—Chair Twists (hold 30 seconds): 2 reps each side Chair Twist (right): slide left leg back to—Lunge Twist (hold 30 seconds) Unwind the body into Triangle (right)—Triangle Flags (hold 30 seconds each): 5 sets Runner's Lunge (right leg forward) grab dumbbells—Knee Floor Kissers (10 reps)—On Your Marks (10 reps)—Plank (hold 30 seconds) Standing Forward Bend Plank—Wrench (1 time each side, hold 30 seconds) Forearm Plank—Plank—Forearm Plank—Plank—Forearm Plank (hold 30 seconds) **Do the whole routine 1-3+ times** **Pick 3 long, deep holds**
NOTES:	

INTERMEDIATE WORKOUT: WEEK 4	
Day 1 & 3	**Day 2 & 4**
Warm-Up Down Dog—Shooting Star (right leg up)—Shooting Star in Motion—Shooting Star—Knee Kissers—Plank—Knee Kissers: 5 sets Plank: hold 30 seconds Chateranga—Upward Dog—Down Dog Repeat on other side Do 3 sets each side, after the third set: Walk to standing 50 Jumping Jacks—50 Take-Offs—Faux Jump Rope (30 seconds) Down Dog—Warrior 2 (right leg forward, hold 30 seconds)—Biceps Curl (while in Warrior 2, 10 reps)—Shoulder Press (10 reps)—Reverse Warrior (hold 30 seconds)—Warrior 2 (hold 30 seconds)—Right Angle (hold 30 seconds)—Fan the Fire (10 reps) Reverse Warrior (hold 30 seconds)—Right Angle (hold 30 seconds)—Fan the Fire (opposite direction, 10 reps)—Warrior 1—Biceps Curl (10 reps) Lunge (hold 30 seconds, grab medicine ball)—Knee Floor Kissers as you Shoulder Press (with medicine ball, 20 reps) Warrior 1—Pinwheels (30 seconds)—Warrior 3—Hold the Bundle (left knee to chest)—Deliver the Bundle (5 reps)—Standing Mountain—Plank Push-Ups (5 reps) Chateranga—Upward Dog—Down Dog Repeat on other side **Do the whole routine 1-3+ times** **Pick 3 long, deep holds**	**Warm-Up** (This whole workout can be done with wrist and ankle weights) Standing Mountain—Standing Forward Bend (hold 30 seconds)—Plank—Wrench (hold 30 seconds, 4 reps each hand)—Chateranga—Upward Dog—Down Dog—Plank—Push-Ups (10 reps) Lower to belly—Locust (10 reps) Canoe (10 reps)—Child's Pose—Boat (hold 30 seconds) Boat-Ins (20 reps, hold medicine ball)—Boat Twists (20 reps, hold medicine ball) Inverted Plank (hold 30 seconds)—Shark Attack (25 reps) Lower to seated Standing Forward Bend—Standing Mountain—Serpentine Jumps (1 minute) Run in place (1 minute)—Butt Kicks (30 seconds) Standing Forward Bend—Plank—Knee Kissers (10 reps each side) Chateranga—Cobra—Cobra Push-Ups (25 reps)—Cobra (hold 1 minute)—Down Dog Down Dog Push-Ups: 25 reps **Do the whole routine 1-3+ times** **Pick 3 long, deep holds**
NOTES:	

INTERMEDIATE WORKOUT: WEEK 5	
Day 1 & 3	**Day 2 & 4**
Warm-Up	**Warm-Up**
Chateranga—Upward Dog—Down Dog (hold 30 seconds) Shooting Star (right leg up)—Shooting Star in Motion—Shooting Star—Down Dog—Table—Clock Holds (right leg, hold 30 seconds)—Down Dog—Runner's Lunge (right leg forward)—Pinwheels (1 minute)—Stop Traffic (hold 1 minute) Eagle Lunge (left arm under right, hold 30 seconds)—Eagle (hold 30 seconds)—Eagle Lunge	Child's Pose—Slither—Cobra—Cobra Push-Ups (10 reps) Locust (10 reps) Face Down Snow Angel (10 reps)—Child's Pose Repeat 3 sets
Crescent Lunge Hammie Curl (10 reps with Eagle arms)—Eagle (hold 30 seconds): 3 sets	Down Dog—Shooting Star (right leg up)—Shooting Star in Motion—Shooting Star—Down Dog Repeat on other leg
Crescent Lunge—Crescent Lunge Twist (hold 30 seconds) Plank (hold 30 seconds)—Knee Kissers (10 reps each side)	Table—Seated Mountain Extended Leg Seated Twist (1 minute)—Stop Traffic (1 minute)—Biceps Curl (10 reps) Hikers (5 reps each leg)—Boat—Boat-Ins (20 reps)
Standing Forward Bend—Standing Mountain—Jumping Jacks (1 minute) Yoga Burpees (3 sets)—Standing Forward Bend—Down Dog—Plank—Side Plank (right, top arm circles, 10 reps, grab dumbbell in left hand)—Amens (10 reps) Half Side Plank—Half Side Plank with Karate Kick (10 reps) Plank—Chateranga—Plank—Chateranga—Upward Dog—Down Dog Repeat whole routine on other side	Plow (hold 30 seconds)—Plow Pedal (1 minute each direction) Straddle Forward Bend (seated, hold 30 seconds)—Kaleidoscopes (10 reps) Bridge—Bridge Lifts (10 reps)—Daddy Long Legs (5 reps each leg)—Camel (hold 30 seconds)—Camel Praise (10 reps)—Quad Crunch (10 reps) Child's Pose—Hero (hold 1 minute)—Table—Down Dog—Standing Forward Bend—Standing Mountain—High Knees (1 minute)—Butt Kicks (1 minute)—Child's Pose
Do the whole routine 1-3+ times	**Do the whole routine 1-3+ times**
Pick 3 long, deep holds	**Pick 3 long, deep holds**
NOTES:	

INTERMEDIATE WORKOUT: WEEK 6	
Day 1 & 3	**Day 2 & 4**
Warm-Up (This whole workout can be done with wrist and ankle weights) Chateranga—Upward Dog—Down Dog—Runner's Lunge (right foot forward, hold 30 seconds)—Runner Lunge—Floor Kissers (10 reps)—Lunge Twist—Crescent Lunge—Crescent Lunge Hammie Curl (3 reps)—Half Hero (right leg extended forward)—Crescent Lunge: 5 sets Warrior 3—Crescent Lunge: 5 sets After last Warrior 3, fold over to Standing Split—Split Kicks (10 reps each side)—Standing Forward Bend—Deadlift (barbell, 10 reps, roll to standing with barbell)—Calf Raise Trio (20 reps each position)—Cross-Kicks (2 minutes)—Side to Side Chair (2 minutes) Standing Forward Bend—Split Kicks (10 reps each leg)—Plank—Chateranga—Upward Dog—Down Dog—Wrench (30 seconds each hand)—Lower to belly—Cobra (hold 1 minute) Repeat the whole routine on the other side **Do the whole routine 1-3+ times** **Pick 3 long, deep holds**	**Warm-Up** (This whole workout can be done with wrist and ankle weights) Run in place (2 minutes)—Wall Squat (1 minute) Toe Balance Squat (20 reps)—Wobbles (5 reps)—Twisted Root Abdominals (20 reps each side)—Wobbles—Standing Forward Bend—Plank—Chateranga—Upward Dog—Down Dog—Down Dog Push-Ups (10 reps) Plank (hold 1 minute)—Knee to Nose (10 reps each side)—Plank—Forearm Plank—Plank: 5 sets Forearm Plank: hold 1 minute Heels Drops (10 reps each side, hold right)—Hips Kisses (10 reps) Heel Drops (10 reps, hold left)—Hip Kisses (10 reps)—Plank—Mountain Climbers (1 minute)—push-ups (10 reps) Down Dog—Down Dog Push-Ups (10 reps)—Standing Forward Bend—Standing Mountain—Step-Ups (10 reps each leg)—Figure 4 Chair (left foot across)—Figure 4 Chair Fold (10 reps, unwind left leg)—Skaters (10 reps)—Standing Forward Bend Repeat from Figure 4 Chair on other side **Do the whole routine 1-3+ times** **Pick 3 long, deep holds**
NOTES:	

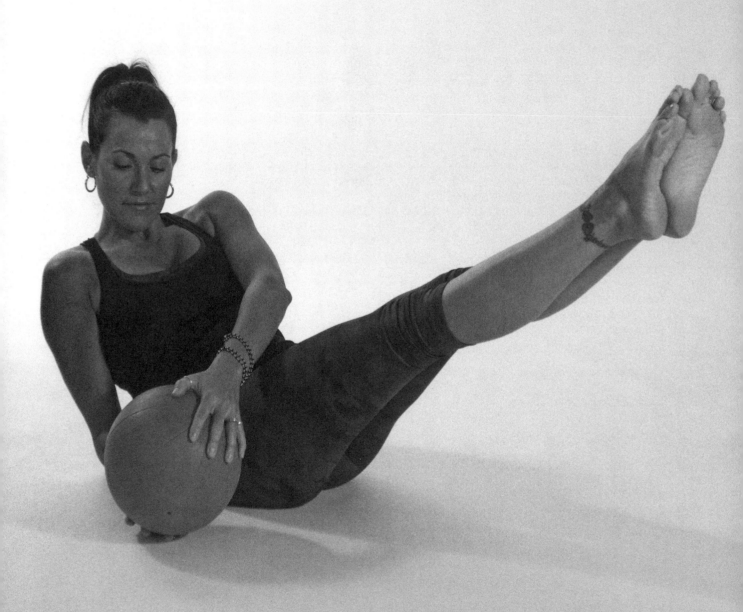

Advanced Workouts

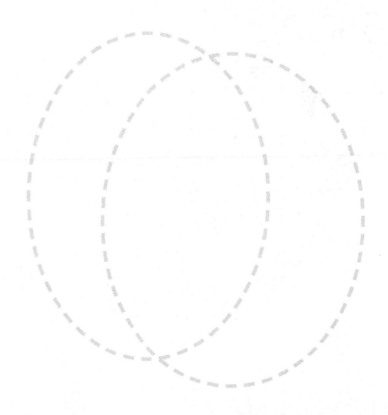

ADVANCED WORKOUT: WEEK 1	
Day 1 & 3	**Day 2 & 4**
Warm-Up	**Warm-Up**
With or without ankle weights (1-2 pounds), wrist weights (1-2 pounds), and weighted vest (5-10 pounds)	**With or without ankle weights (1-2 pounds), wrist weights (1-2 pounds), and weighted vest (5-10 pounds)**
Chateranga—Upward Dog—Down Dog: 5 sets Mountain Climbers (1 minute)—Plank—Heel Drops (20 reps each side)—Knee Kissers (10 each side) Plank—Elbow Me's (right hand, 10 reps)—Elbow Me's (left hand, 10 reps)—Plank Lift right leg and bend the knee—hamstring curl in Plank (10 reps)—Plank—Table Scissors (10 reps) Repeat on other leg Plank—Knee to Nose (right leg, 10 reps)—Plank Cross-Over (10 reps) Switch sides Plank—Side Plank (right)—Plank—Chateranga—Plank—Side Plank (left)—Plank—Chateranga Repeat on other side 3 sets Plank—Plank Cross-Over (10 reps each side)—Standing Forward Bend—Standing Mountain—Rows (10 reps)—Hammer Curl (10 reps)—Faux Jump Rope (1 minute) **Do the whole routine 1-3+ times** **Pick 3 long, deep holds**	Standing Forward Bend—Plank—Chateranga—Upward Dog—Down Dog: 5 sets Standing Mountain—Butt Kicks (1 minute)—High Knees (1 minute)—Standing Forward Bend Warrior 1 (right foot forward, hold 30 seconds)—Runner's Lunge—Lunge Twist (hold 30 seconds)—Warrior 1—Half Hero—Warrior 1—Warrior 3: 5 sets After final Warrior 3: Standing Mountain—Jumping Jacks (1 minute)—Standing Forward Bend—Camel (hold 30 seconds)—Camel Praise (20 reps)—Quad Crunches (20 reps) Plank—Chateranga—lower to belly—Bow (hold 30 seconds)—Locust (hold 30 seconds)—Canoe (10 reps)—Locust (to rest, 10 reps)—Cobra—Cobra Push-Ups (20 reps)—Child's Pose—Slither—Cobra (10 reps) **Do the whole routine 1-3+ times** **Pick 3 long, deep holds**
NOTES:	

ADVANCED WORKOUT: WEEK 2	
Day 1 & 3	**Day 2 & 4**
Warm-Up **With or without ankle weights (1-2 pounds), wrist weights (1-2 pounds), and weighted vest (5-10 pounds)** Standing Forward Bend—Chateranga—Upward Dog—Down Dog Runner's Lunge (right foot forward, hold 30 seconds)—On Your Marks (10 reps)—Knee Floor Kissers (10 reps) Repeat on other side 3 sets each side Runner's Lunge (right foot forward)—SOS (20 reps)—Pinwheels (20 reps)—Lunge Twist (hold 30 seconds) Repeat on other side Standing Straddle Forward Bend—Genies (1 minute)—Straddle Forward Bend (hold 30 seconds)—Triangle (right, hold 30 seconds)—Triangle Flags (hold 30 seconds)—Revolving Triangle (hold 30 seconds)—Standing Straddle Forward Bend Repeat on other side Step to the front of the mat Plank—Chateranga—Upward Dog—Down Dog (hold 30 seconds) Warrior 1 (right foot forward, hold 30 seconds)—Right Angle (hold 30 seconds)—Right Angle Flags (20 reps)—Runner's Lunge—Lunge Twist (hold 30 seconds)—Standing Forward Bend—Cross-Kicks (1 minute)—Spar (30 seconds each side) Repeat on other side Yoga Burpees: 5 sets **Do the whole routine 1-3+ times** **Pick 3 long, deep holds**	**Warm-Up** **With or without ankle weights (1-2 pounds), wrist weights (1-2 pounds), and weighted vest (5-10 pounds)** Standing Forward Bend—Plank—Chateranga—Upward Dog—Down Dog—Runner's Lunge (right foot forward)—Pinwheels (1 minute)—Standing Mountain—Hold the Bundle—Deliver the Bundle (10 reps)—Runner's Lunge Repeat 3 sets Plank—Chateranga—Upward Dog—Down Dog Repeat Runner's Lunge Series on other side Runner's Lunge (right foot forward)—Dragonfly (hold 1 minute)—Plank—Chateranga—Upward Dog—Down Dog Repeat on other side Squat (hold 30 seconds)—Rockets (30 reps)—Take-Offs (20 reps)—Plié Squats (20 reps)—Wobbles (5 reps)—Plow (hold 30 seconds)—Plow Pedal (10 reps each direction)—Shoulder Stand (hold 30 seconds)—Heavy Legs (hold 30 seconds)—Chest Press (in Heavy Legs) (20 reps)—Chest Fly (20 reps)—Tricep Cross Face (20 reps each arm)—Searchlights –(20 reps)—Seals (4 minutes) **Do the whole routine 1-3+ times** **Pick 3 long, deep holds**
NOTES:	

ADVANCED WORKOUT: WEEK 3	
Day 1 & 3	**Day 2 & 4**
Warm-Up **With or without ankle weights (1-2 pounds), wrist weights (1-2 pounds), and weighted vest (5-10 pounds)** **S**tanding Forward Bend—grab weights—Squats (20 reps)—Halfway-Up Flat Back (hold 30 seconds)—Rows (10 reps) Repeat 3 sets Standing Mountain—Jumping Jacks (1 minute)—Faux Jump Rope (1 minute)—Standing Forward Bend—Plank—Yoga Burpees (5 reps) Plank—Chateranga—Upward Dog—Down Dog Half Side Squat (right foot forward, arms up with light weights)—Shoulder Press (10 reps)—Half Side Squat (left foot forward)—Shoulder Press (10 reps)—turn to front—Crescent Lunge (right foot forward, hold 30 seconds)—jump to Crescent Lunge (left foot forward, hold 30 seconds): 3 reps each side—Runner's Lunge (right foot forward)—Lunge Twist (hold 30 seconds)—Plank—Upward Dog—Down Dog Repeat on other side Plank—Squats (20 reps with weights)—Jumping Jacks (1 minute)—Faux Jump Rope (1 minute)—Wobbles (5 reps)—Seated Mountain—Inverted Table (15 reps, hold last Inverted Table 1 minute) Boat (hold 30 seconds)—Boat-Ins (25 reps)—Wobbles—Inverted Plank (hold 1 minute) Rockettes (10 reps each side)—Seated Mountain Biceps Curl (10 reps)—Triceps Extension (10 reps)—Hikers (10 reps each side)—Seated Forward Bend (hold 1 minute) **Do the whole routine 1-3+ times** **Pick 3 long, deep holds**	**Warm-Up** **With or without ankle weights (1-2 pounds), wrist weights (1-2 pounds), and weighted vest (5-10 pounds)** Standing Forward Bend (hold 1 minute with sandbag) Plank—Chateranga—Upward Dog—Down Dog (hold 1 minute) Standing Forward Bend—Split Kicks (10 reps each side) Double Arm Swing: 10 reps Skaters (10 reps each leg)—Hammer Curl (20 reps) Chair (hold 30 seconds)—Standing Forward Bend Repeat 3 sets Chair (hold 30 seconds)—Chair Twist (right, hold 30 seconds)—Chair (hold 30 seconds)—Chair Twist (left, hold 30 seconds)—Chair (hold 30 seconds) Repeat Chair Twist (right)—slide left leg back to Lunge Twist (hold 30 seconds)—Triangle (hold 30 seconds)—Triangle Flags (hold 30 seconds)—Runner's Lunge (grab dumbbells)—Knee Floor Kissers (10 reps)—On Your Marks (10 reps)—Runner's Lunge—Karate Kicks—Runner's Lunge (10 sets) Plank (hold 30 seconds)—Mountain Climbers (30 seconds)—Down Dog—Standing Forward Bend Repeat on other side Plank—Wrench (30 seconds each wrist)—Forearm Plank—Plank—Forearm Plank—Plank—Forearm Plank (hold 1 minute)—Side Forearm Plank (right)—Hip Kisses (10 reps)—Forearm Plank—Side Forearm Plank (left)—Hip Kisses (10 reps) Plank—Down Dog—Standing Forward Bend—Standing Mountain—Jumping Jacks (1 minute)—Butt Kicks (1 minute) **Do the whole routine 1-3+ times** **Pick 3 long, deep holds**
NOTES:	

ADVANCED WORKOUT: WEEK 4	
Day 1 & 3	**Day 2 & 4**
Warm-Up	**Warm-Up**

Day 1 & 3

Warm-Up

With or without ankle weights (1-2 pounds), wrist weights (1-2 pounds), and weighted vest (5-10 pounds)

Down Dog—Shooting Star (right leg)—Shooting Star in Motion—Plank—Knee Kissers (10 reps)—Plank—Elbow Me's (right arm with weight, 10 reps)—Down Dog Push-Ups (5 reps)
Repeat on other side
3 sets each side

Plank (hold 30 seconds)—push-ups (5 reps)—lower to belly—Face Down Snow Angels (5 reps)—Plank—Chateranga—Upward Dog—Down Dog
Repeat on other side
2 sets each side

Down Dog—Warrior 2 (hold 30 seconds)—Biceps Curl (while in Warrior 2, with additional dumbbell, 10 reps)—Shoulder Press (10 reps)—Reverse Warrior (hold 30 seconds)—Warrior 2 (hold 30 seconds)—Front Shoulder Raises (10 reps)—Triceps Extension (10 reps)—Right Angle (hold 30 seconds)—Fan the Fire (10 reps)—Reverse Warrior (hold 30 seconds)—Right Angle—Fan the Fire (10 reps in opposite direction)—Warrior 1—Front Shoulder Raise (10 reps)—Runner's Lunge (hold 30 seconds)—Knee Floor Kissers (hold medicine ball, 10 reps)—Crescent Lunge Twist (hold 30 seconds)—Crescent Lunge—Warrior 3—Runner's Lunge—Pinwheels (1 minute)—Warrior 3—Hold the Bundle (left knee to chest)—Deliver the Bundle (10 reps)—Standing Mountain—Yoga Burpees (3 sets)
Repeat on other side

Plank—Mountain Climbers (1 minute)

Do the whole routine 1-3+ times

Pick 3 long, deep holds

Day 2 & 4

Warm-Up

With or without ankle weights (1-2 pounds), wrist weights (1-2 pounds), and weighted vest (5-10 pounds)

Standing Mountain—Standing Forward Bend—Plank—Wrench (hold 30 seconds, 4 reps each wrist)

Plank Scissors (right leg, 10 reps)—Raise the Roofs (10 reps)
Repeat on other leg
2 sets each leg

Chateranga—Upward Dog—Down Dog—Plank—push-ups (20 reps)—lower to belly Locust (20 reps)—Canoes (25 reps)—Child's Pose—Boat (hold 30 seconds)—Boat-Ins (with medicine ball, 25 reps)—Boat Twists (50 reps alternating)

Inverted Plank—Shark Attacks (25 reps)

Lower to the ground and roll over legs to Standing Forward Bend—Standing Mountain—Serpentine Jumps (1 minute)
Run in place 1 minute—Faux Jump Rope (1 minute)
Standing Forward Bend—grab barbell—Dead Lifts (20 reps)—Plank—Knee Kissers (15 reps each side)—Chateranga—lower to belly—Cobra—Cobra Push-Ups (25 reps)—Cobra (hold 1 minute)—Down Dog—Yoga Burpees (15 sets)

Do the whole routine 1-3+ times

Pick 3 long, deep holds

NOTES:

ADVANCED WORKOUT: WEEK 5	
Day 1 & 3	**Day 2 & 4**
Warm-Up	**Warm-Up**

Day 1 & 3

Warm-Up

With or without ankle weights (1-2 pounds), wrist weights (1-2 pounds), and weighted vest (5-10 pounds)

Chateranga—Upward Dog—Down Dog (hold 30 seconds)
Shooting Star (right leg)—Shooting Star in Motion—Shooting Star—Plank—Knee to Nose (5 reps)—Runner's Lunge—Karate Kick (with left leg)—Runner's Lunge (5 sets)—Pinwheels (1 minute)—Stop Traffic (1 minute)

Grab dumbbells while in Runner's Lunge—Triceps Extension (10 reps)—Hammer Curls (10 reps)—Shoulder Press (10 reps)
Set weights down
Eagle Lunge (left arm under right, hold 30 seconds)—Eagle (hold 30 seconds)—Crescent Lunge (left leg back while in Eagle arms)—Crescent Lunge Hammie Curl (10 reps)—Eagle (hold 30 seconds)—Crescent Lunge—Crescent Lunge Twist (hold 30 seconds)—Plank (hold 30 seconds)—Side to Side Planks (30 seconds)—Knee Kissers (10 reps each side)—Standing Forward Bend—Standing Mountain—Jumping Jacks (1 minute)—Side to Side Chair (1 minute)—Standing Forward Bend—Down Dog

Plank—Side Plank (right)—Side Plank Arm Circles (10 reps)—Amens (10 reps)—Side Plank with Karate Kicks (10 reps)—Cheerleaders (10 reps)—Plank—Side to Side Plank (1 minute)—Chateranga—Upward Dog—Down Dog

Repeat whole routine on other side

Do the whole routine 1-3+ times

Pick 3 long, deep holds

Day 2 & 4

Warm-Up

With or without ankle weights (1-2 pounds), wrist weights (1-2 pounds), and weighted vest (5-10 pounds)

Child's Pose—Slither—Cobra—Cobra Push-Ups (20 reps)
Locust (raise and lower 20 reps)—Face Down Snow Angels (20 reps)—Child's Pose
Repeat 3 sets

Down Dog—Shooting Star (right leg up)—Shooting Star in Motion—Shooting Star—Down Dog
Repeat on other side

Seated Mountain

Extended Leg Seated Twist (1 minute)—Stop Traffic (1 minute)—Biceps Curls (20 reps)—Boat (with medicine ball)—Boat-Ins (1 minute)—Boat Twists (1 minute)—Seated Mountain—Hikers (10 reps each leg)—Boat—Boat-Ins (medicine ball, 20 reps)—Plow—Plow Pedals (1 minute each direction)—Boat—Boat Twists (1 minute)—Seated Mountain—Kaleidoscopes (20 reps)—Bridge—Bridge Lifts (20 reps)—Daddy Long Legs (10 reps each leg)—Camel (hold 30 seconds)—Camel Praise (20 reps)—Quad Crunch (10 reps)—Down Dog—Standing Forward Bend—Standing Mountain—High Knees (1 minute)—Butt Kicks (1 minute)—Run in place 1 minute—Child's Pose

Do the whole routine 1-3+ times

Pick 3 long, deep holds

NOTES:

ADVANCED WORKOUT: WEEK 6	
Day 1 & 3	**Day 2 & 4**
Warm-Up **With or without ankle weights (1-2 pounds), wrist weights (1-2 pounds), and weighted vest (5-10 pounds)** Faux Jump Rope (2 minutes)—Standing Forward Bend—Plank—Chateranga—Upward Dog—Down Dog Runner's Lunge (right leg forward)—Knee Floor Kissers (20 reps)—Lunge Twist (hold 30 seconds)—Crescent Lunge—Crescent Lunge Hammie Curl—Half Hero—Crescent Lunge (3 sets) Warrior 3—Crescent Lunge (5 sets)—after last Warrior 3, Standing Split—alternate Split Kicks (15 reps each side)—Standing Forward Bend—Standing Mountain—kick up to Handstand against wall (hold 1 minute) Standing Back Bend (hold 30 seconds)—Standing Forward Bend—grab barbell—Deadlifts (20 reps)—raise barbell—Shoulder Press (20 reps) Calf Raise Trio (25 reps each position)—Cross-Kicks (2 minutes)—Side to Side Chair (2 minutes)—Plié Squat (1 minute) Standing Forward Bend—Split Kicks (15 reps each leg)—Plank—Chateranga—Upward Dog—Down Dog—Table—Folding Table Cross-Over (15 reps each leg)—Wrench (hold 30 seconds, 3 reps each wrist)—lower to belly Cobra: hold 1 minute Repeat on other side **Do the whole routine 1-3+ times** **Pick 3 long, deep holds**	**Warm-Up** **With or without ankle weights (1-2 pounds), wrist weights (1-2 pounds), and weighted vest (5-10 pounds)** Run in place 1 minute—Wall Squat (1 minute) Toe Balance Squat: 20 reps (hold medicine ball) Wobbles (5 reps)—Twisted Root Abdominals (25 reps each side) Wobbles—Standing Forward Bend—Plank—Chateranga—Upward Dog—Down Dog—Down Dog Push-Ups (25 reps)—Plank (hold 1 minute)—Raise the Roofs (15 reps each side) Plank—Forearm Plank—Plank—Forearm Plank—Plank—Forearm Plank (hold 1 minute) Side Forearm Plank (right)—Hip Kisses (15 reps) Repeat on other side Mountain Climbers: 1 minute Plank—push-ups (10 reps)—Plank—Down Dog—Down Dog Push-Ups (20 reps)—Standing Forward Bend—Step-Ups (15 reps each leg, on bench with dumbbells in each hand)—Standing Mountain—Figure 4 Chair (left foot across)—Figure 4 Chair Folds (10 reps)—Skaters (left leg back, 10 reps) Repeat from Figure 4 Chair on other side Standing Forward Bend—Standing Mountain **Do the whole routine 1-3+ times** **Pick 3 long, deep holds**
NOTES:	

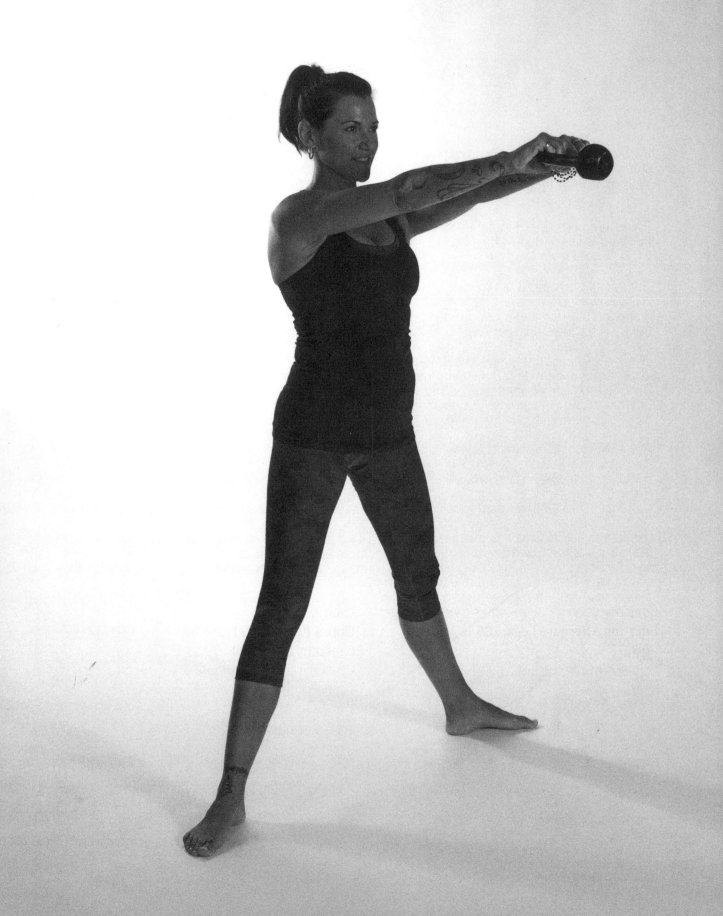

Index of Exercises

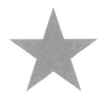

GOT QUESTIONS?
NEED ANSWERS?
GO TO:

GETFITNOW.COM
IT'S FITNESS 24/7

VIDEOS - WOROUTS- FORUMS
ONLINE STORE

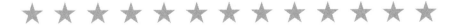